The
Original Diet™

The Omnivore's Solution

Designed by Nature
Researched by a Rocket Scientist

Roy Mankovitz, BS, JD, CNC

Montecito Wellness LLC
Santa Barbara

Notices

The information contained in this book is based upon the research and personal experience of the author. It is not intended as a substitute for consulting with your physician or other healthcare providers. If you choose to follow any of the ideas in this book, you might want to consider first consulting with your doctor about the appropriateness of these suggestions for your particular situation. Nature, not the author, is responsible for any positive (or adverse) effects or consequences resulting from the use of the suggestions or procedures discussed in this book.

Portions of the material presented in this book are the subject of US and foreign issued patents and pending patent applications. No license is granted to the purchaser or reader of this book or to any other individual or entity to commercially or otherwise exploit or offer to others any of these inventions, some of which are listed in Appendix A of this book. The following are trademarks of the author or publisher, or used under license: The Original Diet™, The Wellness Project™, The Original Diet™, Hypothesis for Health™, A Rocket Scientist's Blueprint for Health™, The Dirt Diet™, Officizer™, CellFrame™, Clayodine™, HealthBra™, ABC Food Test™, The Dirt Detox Protocol™, The Mercury-Yeast Spectrum Disorder™, and Whispers of Wisdom®.

Published by:

Montecito Wellness LLC
1482 East Valley Road, Suite 808
Santa Barbara, CA 93108

info@montecitowellness.com
www.montecitowellness.com

ISBN: 978-0-9801584-7-2

Dedication

To my mother Sarah for giving me life, to my wife Kathleen, my children Jill, Alan, Miriam, and Andrea, my grandchildren Alexa and Jordyn, and my sister Toby for their patience and support, and to my father Benjamin and my uncle Solomon, both of whom had their lives cut short as a result of medical errors.

Acknowledgements

In the field of medicine, I wish to acknowledge Dr. Orion Truss, Dr. John Trowbridge, Dr. Broda Barnes, Dr. William Jefferies, Dr. Laszlo Belenyessy, Dr. Hans Gruenn and his wife Annika, Dr. Deitrich Klinghardt, Dr. Michael Gershon, Dr. Guy Abraham, Dr. David Brownstein, Dr. Jorge Flechas, Dr. Paul Dantzig, Dr. Mildred Seelig, Dr. C. Norman Shealy, and Dr. Lawrence Wilson for their courage in pursuing alternative approaches to research and healing. In the field of dentistry, I wish to acknowledge Dr. Weston A. Price, Dr. George Meinig, Dr. Hal Huggins, Dr. David Villarreal, and Leo Cashman for their courage in pursuing alternative approaches to treatment. In the field of anthropology, I wish to acknowledge Vilhjalmur Stefansson, Jared Diamond, and Cindy Engel for their pioneering studies, which opened many windows into our past. In the field of cellular biology, I wish to acknowledge Dr. Leslie Wilson and Dr. George Ayoub of the University of California at Santa Barbara for their research skills and support. In the field of emotional detoxification, I would like to acknowledge Bert Hellinger, JoAnna Chartrand, and Dyrian Benz for their work in healing the psyche. Last but not least, I wish to acknowledge the support of John Posa, Esq., and Dr. Julie Staple, Esq.

Contents

Prologue

Close friends often refer to me as a disruptive innovator, meaning that I tend to create, invent, develop, or otherwise come up with ideas that upset the *status quo* in a variety of disciplines. I tend not to be satisfied with merely accepting on faith what others have determined to be the solution to a particular problem. I love research, and make it a habit to learn whatever I can in an area of interest, and then see if I can step back and approach the problem in a different way, often replacing the old with something new and hopefully improved. From a definition point of view, a disruptive innovation is one that improves or changes a product or service in ways that the market does not expect. A disruptive innovation ignores the currently popular paradigms and creates new ones.

Historically, I have repeated this disruptive process in a number of disciplines. When I began my career in the field of rocket science, the traditional approach to modeling the behavior of spacecraft was to use analog computers as the tool of choice. I chose to replace the analog computer by emulating its behavior on a digital computer, and then proceeding from there. Some of the results of this disruptive behavior are listed in Appendix A of this book under my various NASA publications.

My entry into the commercial world of electronics was based on a bold statement that I had made to the president of a company that made electromechanical switches called relays. I told him these switches were not sufficiently reliable for use in long space journeys and other critical applications because they contained moving parts that could eventually wear out from extended use. I told him that if I had the time, I could develop an equivalent switch that had no moving parts, and hence not wear out. He hired me to do just that, and the result was the formation of a new industry that produces solid state relays and circuit breakers to replace the old versions in critical applications. Some of my patents in this area are also listed in Appendix A.

When I entered the world of consumer electronics, it was with the intent of simplifying the VCR recording of TV shows by consumers. That project spawned a feature known as VCR Plus that was built into virtually every VCR to simplify the recording process by replacing the old one which was too complicated. Along the way, I assisted in developing the on-screen television guide, widely available from most cable companies, to replace the print guide provided in newspapers. Now, those electronic guides make it even easier to record programs using a digital recorder. A list of my patents in this area are also in Appendix A, along with those devoted to making radio listening an interactive experience, a feature yet to be deployed by the broadcast industry.

In the field of intellectual property law, I chose to implement a different model aimed at protecting and monetizing the patent rights of companies and individuals, spawning an entire industry devoted to doing just that.

Being a disruptive innovator has its rewarding moments, when something new replaces something old in a manner that yields an improvement that is appreciated by those who benefit from that improvement. Then, there is the other side of the coin – those who are being disrupted by the new – the disruptees. By way of example, how do you think the buggy-whip manufacturers felt toward Henry Ford? You get the idea – the disruptees can get downright upset about some new idea replacing their cherished businesses (or beliefs), even if the overall result is an eventual benefit to society.

Well, with that as background, it now brings me to the field of health and the art of medicine, areas that have held great interest for me over the last several decades. The first book I published on the subject is entitled *The Wellness Project – A Rocket Scientist's Blueprint for Health*. It includes a discussion of how I first became interested in health, how I became disenchanted with the information and counseling I was receiving from those trained in the subject, how I started over to re-research the area using the skills I had previously developed, and the startling, unexpected, and clearly disruptive conclusions that emerged from this twenty year project. Not surprisingly, readers are primarily divided into two groups. The first group has been extremely supportive of the novel hypotheses and conclusions I have drawn (backed by hundreds of references), which in many instances are in opposition to the firmly entrenched beliefs of those in the medical, dental and alternative heath fields. This group includes very open-minded and prominent MDs, dentists, and psychotherapists, as well as people from all walks of life who have been looking for unbiased answers in these fields, based on common sense and humility. The second group includes the unhappy disruptees, some of whom make their livelihood supporting the entrenched approaches to health, whether they are mainstream or alternative, and some of whom are consumers who do not want to challenge the *status quo*, since doing so may undermine their fundamental belief system as it applies to health and the medical establishment.

I am in the fortunate position that I do not have to make a living in the health or medical fields, allowing me a totally unbiased view. My motivation for writing books in this field is in the hope that I can help at least some readers with their health problems, and I get great joy when I find that such is the case. Profits made from the sale of my books go back into funding additional research in the fields of wellness and illness prevention.

Now, about this book, *The Original Diet – The Omnivore's Solution*. It is excerpted from the diet sections of my previously published book, *The Wellness Project – A Rocket Scientist's Blueprint for Health [1]*. That book goes into great detail describing my history and research as applied to an overall wellness plan, including diet, detoxification, and lifestyle programs designed to reverse illness and maintain health. Some readers indicated to me that it was too much information to assimilate, and that they were primarily only interested in the eating plans, or primarily only interested in the detox and lifestyle (healthy environment) plans. To accommodate them, I created this book for those interested in the diet plans, and created another book, *Nature's Detox Plan – A Program for Physical and Emotional Detoxification[2]* , which is derived from the detox and lifestyle sections of *The Wellness Project*, to accommodate readers whose interests lie in those areas.

Section One - The Hypothesis for Health

Common sense is not so common - Voltaire

The diet program in this book is not based on dispensing drugs or supplements to be taken for a lifetime. It is not a weight loss program; it is not an exercise program; it is neither symptom nor diagnosis based. In a nutshell, it is designed to use food to restore a human body as closely as possible to the condition intended by Nature, to the extent our current knowledge allows. It uses very simple principles, including common sense and humility, to produce a program designed to yield positive results.

The theory that underlies the Original Diet is that if a person eats foods that they are not adapted to eat because of their unique ancestral history, their body's defense system will react to those foods as toxins, and mount a defense against them. If your defense system, which I define as a combination of your immune system and any other parts of your body designed to maintain your health, is busy detoxifying your food three or more times per day, it does not leave much left over to protect you from serious illnesses such as cancer and heart disease. Overworking the defense system can also lead to its malfunction, where it attacks what appear to be health tissues, leading to a whole list of autoimmune conditions such as arthritis, lupus, and others.

In today's environment, a great deal of the foods available to us were certainly not available to our ancestors, and hence some of these foods may not be healthy for us to eat. The question I attempt to answer in this book is: what are the right foods for each of us that will contribute to our health, as opposed to disrupting it? There is no doubt in my mind that there are plenty of people out there who have acquired, probably by random chance, the evolutionary makeup that fits our modern food environment. These are the *winners* in our environment, individuals that seemingly can eat anything, smoke, drink, get little sleep, never exercise, work in a toxic environment, and live a perfectly healthy symptom-free life into triple digit years. How do you know if you are one of the *winners* in our present day Western society? You have no aches or pains, lots of energy, a cheery disposition, no illnesses, radiant skin, no weight problems, take no medications, eat whatever you want, and can't understand why others don't share your good fortune.

One of the difficulties in determining what foods are compatible with our particular ancestral background, which includes our genetic makeup, is that many of us do not know with any degree of certainty our heritage from both sides of our family. Further, there is every likelihood that, through many generations of intermarriage, we are a melting pot of different heritages. Compound that with anthropological studies showing that our ancestors have roamed the Earth for about 2.5 million years (about 100,000 generations), and we have a serious task ahead of us.

One of the simplest of questions I had been trying to get answered over the last twenty-five years from the healthcare community was "What should I eat to prevent illness and keep myself healthy"? After all, knowing what to eat can't be as difficult as rocket science! Since foods can be a source of toxins, and we usually eat three times per day, eating the wrong foods could add up to a very large load on the defense system. So, I needed the right answers, and I made it my first goal to find out what foods would be in alignment with my evolutionary history, and hence would prove lowest in potential toxins.

I consulted with many nutritionists, and each gave me a different answer. Out of frustration, I read every book I could find on nutrition, and studied for and passed a test to become certified as a nutritional consultant. However, neither the books on health nor the certification brought me any closer to finding my answers. In fact, I was somewhat alarmed to realize that the "science of nutrition" lacked the rigors of my field that enabled rockets to get off the launch pad, and DVD players to work. Did you know that there is no agreed upon definition for the words *fruit, vegetable, nut, seed,* or *bean* – or even the term *Vitamin E*; that we do not know the complete composition of any food or how these various food elements interact with each other in the body; that we have not identified the majority of friendly bacteria in our gut that are critical to digestion and keep us alive; or that we only recently discovered that our gut has its own nervous system that can act independently of our brain; or that the gut produces more serotonin than our brain and can have a major impact on our emotions [3]? Keep this in mind the next time you have a "gut feeling" about something.

It took me twenty years of independent research to find the right answers, and now that I am a nutritionist, I feel comfortable answering the question for others and myself. It is an answer unlike any given to me by those who are supposed to have the answers, is one I had never seen in print before, and it forms the starting point for The Original Diet. Guess what? There is one particular diet that all humans originally evolved to eat, just as other species of mammals have a diet that has uniquely evolved to keep them healthy.

Please note carefully that the previous sentence does not state there is *only one* diet for each individual that must be followed to produce health. In fact, there may be many diets each person can adopt that will yield an illness-free life. I will provide guidelines so that the reader can experiment with different foods in an intelligent manner, guided by clues from Nature which, for the most part, we have come to ignore. My point is that among these various dietary choices, there appears to be one in particular (I will call it the Original Diet) that is safe for every person to eat, based on our common human heritage. This is a very subtle but important point. Here is a simple analogy. All modern gasoline engine powered cars can run smoothly and safely on 91-octane fuel. Some can also run smoothly and safely on 89-octane fuel, or perhaps some form of biogas. If you were given such a car with no operating instructions, the safe thing to do would be to fill it with 91-octane fuel, rather than risk using the wrong stuff. As you read this book, you will see the importance of this simple analogy as it relates to the entire field of nutrition and dietary choices.

I refer to our ancestors often in this book because that is where I finally found the answers I was looking for. I am not referring to the "ancient" Greeks or Romans or Egyptians, or Eastern medicine such as Ayurveda, or Biblical times or Aztecs or Mayans. I found my answers before any of these (or written language, or farms, or villages, or towns, or empires) were in existence. Humans have been roaming the Earth for about 2.5 million years, and all of the above took place within the last 5000 to 10000 years, so none of what we normally think of as ancient is really ancient at all.

As you will see, to get the answers I needed, I went back in time before fire was used for cooking, estimated to be somewhere between

20,000 and 150,000 years ago (800 to 6000 generations ago), defined as the Paleolithic era (I will abbreviate it as Paleo in the book). But isn't it true that our ancestors way back then lived short lives because of illness, and also had high infant mortality? No, that is not true. Incredibly, our Paleo Ancestors of that time (from skeletal evidence) were on average taller than we are today, had bone strength higher than ours, and had virtually perfect teeth, all strong indicators of robust health. Paleontologists believe that our early ancestors would have lived long healthy lives except for three things: starvation, predators, and accidents, none of which has anything to do with illness [4-7]. Take away your supermarket; put yourself in a wild animal park; and suffer an arm or leg fracture; and you too would be challenged to reach a nice, ripe old age. If there was a high infant mortality back then (we have no evidence that there was), the odds of us being here today would be quite slim.

From my research in anthropology and Paleopathology, it actually appears that our species reached its pinnacle of health somewhere around 10,000 years ago (400 generations). Something happened in the last 400 generations to reverse this course and take us backward and downward. These "somethings" will be discussed below. Out of my studies came the framework for The Original Diet. The concept is to use Nature as the template for bringing our current lifestyle into alignment with our evolutionary heritage at that time in the past when we were so healthy. The premise is that if we perform such an alignment, our body will return to and stay at a pinnacle of health with an unburdened defense system. Unfortunately, the "height" of the health pinnacle for each of us is not readily predictable, because it is affected by many personal variables including certain genetic defects, as well as permanent damage to and removal of important body parts, discussed in more detail below.

The Original Diet is based on the largest health "study" ever conducted in the history of our species. It extended over a period of about 2.4 million years (about 96,000 generations), involved millions of our ancestors, and flies in the face of virtually every health program written to date.

Chapter 1 – A Search for Answers

Be careful about reading health books. You may die of a misprint!- Mark Twain

During my engineering career, I worked with many smart folks at the Jet Propulsion Laboratory, a NASA facility operated by the California Institute of Technology, designing unmanned spacecraft control systems. I am a named inventor in more than 60 U.S. patents and hundreds of corresponding foreign patents (please see Appendix A). I have additional patent applications pending in the U.S. Patent and Trademark Office, some of which are in the field of health, and I will tell you more about a few of them later in the book. I come to the health field with an engineer's and inventor's perspective, and since the body is really a complex chemical factory, these skills work very effectively to help me devise methods to try to understand it. Here are some of the analogies I used.

If I was presented with a complex device (my body) that did not have accompanying operating instructions, and I wanted to find out how it was designed to work, I would have several alternatives. A first approach very familiar to engineers is called "reverse engineering," where we endeavor to take the device apart, ideally without damaging it, so that we can compare its inner workings with our prior knowledge in order to try and figure it out. A second approach that we are all familiar with from our consumer electronics experiences is to just start pushing buttons somewhat randomly and see what happens. (Sometimes we do this even though we were given operating instructions!) This approach is commonly called a "trial and error" approach. A third approach is to contact the manufacturer and communicate directly with the person or team that designed the device. I don't know of a name for this approach so I will make one up: I will call it the "common sense" approach, and as you will see, it forms the backbone of the eating plans. So, let's look at each of these approaches as they apply to the human effort to understand how we are designed to work. The presumption is that if we had this understanding, we would be well along the road to maintaining ourselves in a state of health.

Considering the first approach of reverse engineering, it is believed that somewhere about 300 BCE, Herophilus, referred to as the Father of Anatomy, began dissecting cadavers and documenting what he saw. These crude endeavors continued over the next 1000 years or so to provide us with an anatomical road map that allows skilled surgeons to put us back together when our parts are damaged. Unfortunately, this technique has yet to produce any useful results in finding the causes of the major chronic illnesses that plague us today.

Now, let's explore the second, or button-pushing approach to finding out how our body is designed to work. I will hereafter refer to this as the "trial and error" (T&E) approach, which is actually a form of experiment. As we will see, this approach is the mainstay of the healthcare industry in its efforts to treat illness, from the development of new drugs or supplements to creating treatment protocols.

I love electronic gadgets, and am an avid button-pusher, which has gotten me into no end of trouble. In many cases, I either have to resort to reading the instructions (drat!) or, as a final resort, calling the manufacturer to get the answer as to how to restore the gadget to its proper operating condition. Some manufacturers, bless their heart, provide a button on their widget that can be used as a factory reset – if only we humans had such a feature! Personally, my button-pushing behavior can be characterized as somewhat motivated by a sense of arrogance- I don't need anyone to tell me how this thing works, I can figure it out myself!

From a study of the theory of evolution and of the history of our present human species, it is apparent that Nature makes great use of T&E experiments in evolving species. It seems to work like this: random mutations and genetic and probably other variations occur all the time in every species and these can be viewed as the *trials*, while poor reproductive fitness is regarded as the *error*. Thus after long periods of time, well-adapted evolutionary patterns accumulate simply by virtue of their being able to reproduce, while less well-adapted patterns die out. Now "die out" can be a euphemism for many different behaviors, from a failure to reproduce to debilitating birth defects to chronic illness, but the end result is the cessation of that line of evolutionary patterns. So in a

T&E experiment run by Nature, a failure is clearly demarcated and is not perpetuated indefinitely.

At about ten to twelve thousand years ago (about 400 generations ago), we gained sufficient intelligence and had developed enough tools to begin some very serious T&E "button pushing" ourselves with respect to virtually all aspects of our lives. Not only that, the scope of these T&E experiments was substantially increased because of the development of societies that were grouped into towns and villages, so that one experiment could effect very large numbers of people. As you will see, humans have conducted experiments that have not only fooled with Nature, but have reversed many of the biological gains made in our health up to that time.

For the human evolutionary period older than 400 generations ago, (a period of about 2.49 million years, or 99,600 generations), it is believed by many in the field of anthropology that our ancestors, living primarily in tropical Africa, led a nomadic life consisting of hunting and gathering. I will refer to this period as the Ancient or Paleo Era (see the side box entitled Defining Ancient for further clarification), and the more recent period following the Paleo Era as the Neolithic era.

The T&E experiments during the Paleo era would have included Nature fiddling with mutations and other variations, the results of which may have taken a very long time to surface (perhaps several hundred thousand years); and some simple experiments devised by humans, such as sampling new sources of food.

The T&E system works very well for humans when the E follows soon after the T, so that a cause and effect relationship can be established. Push the wrong button and the screen goes blank. Eat the wrong food and you soon get sick. In these experiments one quickly learns (and hopefully teaches others) to avoid that behavior. Animals do that all the time with eating and other behavior and, in ways we do not understand, pass a lot of that information on to their offspring. A problem with humans running T&E experiments on themselves is our relatively short lifespan (perhaps 120 years maximum) compared to our 2.5 million year evolutionary heritage. Eating something and getting sick an hour later is a no-brainer, but how about eating something that does not show its damage for a decade, or for three generations, or for 400 generations?

Defining Ancient

The word Ancient has many meanings in the field of health. In this book, the term refers to a prehistoric era distinguished by the development of stone tools. It covers the greatest portion of humanity's time on Earth, extending from about 2.5 million years ago, with the introduction of stone tools to the introduction of fire for cooking, estimated at around 100,000 years ago. **THE TERM "ANCIENT" <u>DOES NOT</u> REFER TO THE FOLLOWING, ALL OF WHICH ARE RELATIVELY <u>MODERN</u>:**

Biblical Times	Any Empire or Dynasty
Roman Times	Greek Times
Egyptian Times	Large city or town
Ayurveda/Eastern Medicine	Farms
Yoga	Ranches
Tai Chi	Growing of crops
Domestication of animals	Harvesting
Mayans/Incas	Polynesians
American Indians	Inuits

The problem is compounded by the fact that the human body is not a static device like most human made things, but is alive and constantly evolving, renewing, healing, and adapting to its environment. This is coupled with the fact that we humans continue to run multiple T&E experiments in parallel, in many cases not even realizing these are experiments. (Those of us who like to run experiments know that this behavior is disastrous, leading to chaos and conclusions that are wrong.) All of this is going on during the interval between starting the Trial and recognizing the Error, so that when the Error is finally recognized (if at all), it may be impossible to link it to the correct cause (or combination of causes). Sound like a nightmare? It is, and unfortunately it also could be said to characterize our progress in health (or lack thereof) over the last 400 generations. In the following chapters, I will touch upon examples of what I (and some others) regard as faulty T&E experiments carried out by our fellow humans (many times in good faith), some as far back as 10,000 years ago, that are now manifesting as chronic illnesses for many of us.

Let's go on to the third approach (common sense) to finding out how we were designed to work. As you may recall, this approach was to contact the manufacturer of the widget in hopes of communicating with the designer/engineer or team thereof to get the real scoop on how the widget works and how to keep it working that way for as long as possible. Well, "who" or "what" designed us? While I am certainly aware of the faith-based answers to this question, in this book, I refer to our designer as Nature. While I would like to have a side box defining what I mean by the term Nature, I am at a loss for words. The best I can come up with is this: Nature is that which has caused everything in our universe (and probably others) to evolve and exist. Because of our human conceptual limitations, it is much easier to give Nature human attributes in our attempt at definition. So, when I make statements such as Nature does this or that, or Nature intended ...., it is really a combination of ignorance and arrogance on my part. I cannot ultimately "know" what Nature was or is "doing" or "intending", and it is arrogant of me to think that I do know. However, this is the best I can do, so please bear with me.

So, what happens since Nature has not provided us with written operating instructions? Well, in the animal kingdom, a great deal of knowledge is passed from generation to generation regarding what to eat and how to self heal [8]. Since we are also part of the animal kingdom, I presume such information was also passed along in the human chain, but somehow got lost along the way. A large portion of this book is devoted to efforts to reconstruct this lost knowledge to the greatest extent possible, and then to apply what we have learned to our modern lifestyle – this is the derivation of The Original Diet, the starting point for our eating programs. The goal is to do as good a job as possible to align our environment to our heritage, with the expectation that by doing so we are capitalizing on the successful result of 99,600 generations of Nature's Trial and Error experiments. If one believes the Darwinian model of evolution, then, but for our own interference in Nature's experiments, we now should be at a very high pinnacle of health, having had 100,000 replication cycles to discard untold numbers of failed evolutionary experiments in favor of the ones that produce optimum wellbeing.

I am certainly not alone in believing that a "return to Nature" would be a healthy thing to do as compared with where most of us are now. In furtherance of this goal, several studies have been conducted in the field of anthropology to try to deduce what our Paleo Ancestors ate [9], and yet others have studied modern hunter-gatherer societies to try to determine their lifestyle and its effects on health [6]. Still others have investigated the effects of domestication on the health of our pets [10], from which we can deduce some interesting information about our own diets.

Before we move on to the next chapter, I suspect that some readers may continue to take exception to the premise that our Ancient ancestors were healthy or that they should be viewed as a model for us. Why, isn't it true that they rarely lived past 30 or so, certainly not long enough to have gotten the chronic diseases like cancer, atherosclerosis, and diabetes generally associated with aging? Weren't their lives nasty, brutish, and short? Or how about this argument: Nature has no use for us after our reproductive years are over. Although we will address these issues in more depth in later chapters, this is a good place for a sanity check.

Let's try to find some common sense answers to these questions: First, the way evolution works, at least in the animal kingdom, (barring human interference) is that with few exceptions species evolve over time to become stronger, not weaker, and experts such as UCLA environmental historian and Pulitzer Prize winning author Jared Diamond discount statements to the contrary. As mentioned earlier, these experts argue that our early ancestors would have lived long healthy lives except for three things: starvation, predators, and accidents (none of which has anything to do with illness).

As I already mentioned, our Paleo Ancestors of about 400 generations ago were on average taller than we are today, had bone strength higher than ours, and had virtually perfect teeth, all indicators of robust health. As we shall see in the following chapters, something happened in the last 400 generations to reverse this course and take us backward and downward. Oh, regarding the ditty that Nature has no use for us after reproductive years, it is somewhat well established that Nature has endowed our cells with about a 120-year life, and that male humans have reproductive capacity their entire lives. So, if this idea made any sense, males would far outlive females (they do not), who (for reasons we do not understand) run out of eggs way before 120.

It has puzzled me as to why it is so well entrenched in our culture that our ancestors led short lives filled with illness and high infant mortality. Where did these stories come from? Well it finally occurred to me that they were referring to a different group of our ancestors, and this is the reason I went to the trouble of defining the term Ancient with a capital A. There is no question that the so-called ancient civilizations, such as the Egyptians, Greeks and Romans and their successors did indeed live short lives prone to illness and high infant mortality, and that is what these stories are referring to. Because we expect, rightly so, that each generation would be healthier than the previous, which is the way Nature works when undisturbed, it is counterintuitive to think that our ancestors living before these civilizations could possibly have been healthier than later generations, but that is the case. It is why I finally abandoned research into the so-called "ancient" medical wisdom of the Greeks and Romans and the Far East Dynasties, none of which are truly Ancient. Why should I dwell on this body of knowledge when the generations before them were much healthier? In my opinion, the Ancient time period is where the real health pearls of wisdom lie and, sure enough, that is what I found.

My research is based on what could be considered the largest "clinical trial" in the history of the human species, having been conducted and refined over a period of about 2.49 million years, and involving millions of our ancestors. Until recently, (about 10,000 years ago) the results of these trials, from a health point of view, were a great success, which is why our species exists today. It allowed our ancestors over most of the last two-and-a-half million years to survive in a quite healthy fashion. This survival over eons has much to offer contemporary man who has strayed far from Nature's blueprint and who, despite the marvels of modern sanitation, medicine, and technology, wallows in chronic illness.

The ideas contained on these pages reflect my experience, an attempt to reconnect with Nature's fundamentals for the sake of my

health. I invite you to consider the ideas as possible tools for your own
health.

How To Use This Book

In the chapter that follows, I document what I call Faulty Human
Trials – a list of some Trial & Error experiments concocted by humans in
the area of nutrition over the last 400 generations and foisted on virtually
all of civilization.   These experiments are ongoing today, and in my
humble opinion, either singly or in combination, contribute to the causes
of virtually all chronic illnesses because of their potential to produce
toxins in the body. I complete the chapter by disclosing how some of
these experiments adversely affected my own life and how, by "opting out"
of the experiments and going back in time to a prior point, I have been
able to restore and maintain my health.

Regard this book as a nutritional blueprint for better health, and
not a cookbook with recipes. I will lay out my theories of how our
heritage developed when we allowed Nature to be in charge. These
suggestions can have a powerful effect, and they helped me achieve relief
from many annoying symptoms, giving me the ability to rise to a higher
level of health. The sincere intention of my hypothesis is illness
prevention, and for those already ill, the reversal of the condition. The
approach is really a "one-size-fits-all" set of ideas based on alignment with
Nature. They are designed to benefit the body regardless of specific
symptoms or illnesses, such as cancer or diabetes or Parkinson's or acne.

Chapter 2 - Fooling (With) Mother Nature

It's not nice to fool Mother Nature! -
1970s Margarine Commercial

I like the concept of "Mother Nature." Somehow, I find it comforting to think of our designer in feminine terms – soft, comforting, and nurturing. Of course, She does exhibit some behavior that seems out of character – earthquakes, hurricanes, drought, a tiger taking down an antelope and tearing it to pieces. My point is that there are some things we like about Nature and others we do not and would like to change or at least control. We have an inkling about how She works (our so-called Laws of Nature), but for the most part we are quite clueless.

I would like to keep my writing style in this book as gender-neutral as possible, trying to avoid terms like Paleo Man and Mother Nature, so here is a shot at it. I will sometimes refer to our Paleo Ancestor as "PA," and to Mother Nature as "MA," with the caveat that we owe our existence to the fact that PA paid a great deal of attention to MA!

As a techno-geek, I have had an inflated sense that I understand how things work. I get a great deal of satisfaction in inventing and making things that perform, but these are not living things. My research into health has really humbled me. I have read many of the same texts used in medical schools, and it has opened my eyes as to how truly little we know about the world of *living things*. I now know that there is no way in my lifetime that I will be able to understand the workings of nature in sufficient detail to reproduce a living thing from scratch, or even to modify the way my body works in ways that Nature did not intend, without the possibility of causing harm. So, my best bet is to try to find out what Nature did intend for me, and to stick to it as closely as possible. The real beauty of this approach is that I do not have to understand *why* we evolved to eat certain foods or follow a particular lifestyle, or even to understand how the body works – it is enough just to know the plan. This is an enormous relief and allows me to concentrate on preparing the blueprint for wellness, which is really Nature's blueprint, not mine. My task is to figure it out as best as possible and document it.

The reason I have spent the last few paragraphs dwelling on Nature is in preparation for a discussion of what I consider to be some major experiments directly affecting our health. These are in the form of Trial & Error experiments in nutrition conducted by humans over the last 10,000 years (and still going on today) that undoubtedly had and continue to have a major negative impact on the health of a significant portion of the population by directly or indirectly raising the body's toxin burden. One can look at these experiments as attempts to fool or change Mother Nature in ways that are supposed to provide a benefit to our species that Nature has not provided. In my opinion, we may fool *with* Nature (that is, we have the *ability* to launch these experiments), but to think that in our lifetime, or even over a hundred generations, we can actually cause Nature to modify her plan for us, evolved over 2.5 million years, is somewhat unrealistic. To remind myself of my relationship with Nature, I periodically go to the beach and walk out into the ocean, positioning myself squarely in front of a large breaking wave – very humbling.

Ten Thousand Years of Human Experiments

Referring to Table 1, I have listed what I consider to be some of the major experiments in nutrition conducted by humans over the last 400 or so generations, which have the potential of adversely affecting our health and are moving some of us (the *others*) down the road to illness. However, for many of the *winners* in our society, some of the items on this list would not be viewed as a problem at all, because they have little or no negative impact on their health. For the rest of us, some of these Trial & Error experiments have proved faulty because their intended outcome, while initially designed to improve our lives, is causing or contributing to illness in our body by increasing its toxic load. In many instances, we have yet to recognize that fact, or if we do recognize it, to take the necessary action to stop it. One reason for our lack of recognition is the long interval between the start of the trial and the manifestation of the error, so that we have lost track of the cause/effect relationship. As part of this problem, we have also lost the reference point or baseline that we started with, leaving us with meaningless comparisons to arbitrary reference points. Another reason is our lack of knowledge of how the body works, leaving us clueless as to how a cause could possibly result in a particular effect.

I have limited the list (which if it included all of the ecological insults to us and our environment, would have gone on for pages) to those items that are somewhat under our control as individuals and that can be either changed or at least dealt with personally through reasonable effort, and which affect large segments of society. In Section 2 of this book I will briefly discuss each, touching on the motivation for the experiment, the impact it has had on humans, and at least one way to "opt out" of it. In a way, this is an attempt to return to Nature's evolutionary experiment, picking up where we left off before we meddled with the plan.

Table 1
Ten Thousand Years of Fooling With Mother Nature
A Partial List of Potentially Faulty Human Trials Related to Nutrition

Eating Grains	Fluoridation
Eating Dairy/Pasteurization	Plastic Food Containers
Eating Concentrated Sugars	Microwaving Food
Feeding Unnatural Food to our Food	Infant Formulas
	Ingesting Ice
Eating Plants Protected by Nature	Chlorinated Water
Artificial Sweeteners	

As I mentioned before, all of these are ongoing experiments, so one must assume that somebody considers them worthwhile. These "somebodies" are very powerful entities indeed, including virtually the entire Western and Eastern health and dental communities (including a substantial portion of the alternative health industry), as well as food, cosmetic and chemical industries (and governments and universities) worldwide. They certainly do not consider the items on my list as faulty, since in many cases they form the backbone of their businesses or are major contributors to their income. There really is no money in discrediting the items on this list. To the contrary, there is enormous money at stake to perpetuate these experiments.

Chapter 3 - An Overview of the Project

Life in all its Fullness is Mother Nature Obeyed

– Weston A. Price

The discussion that follows could be thought of as a roadmap that can be followed by individuals to improve their heath based on their choice of foods to eat. As mentioned earlier, the hypothesis behind the program states that by increasing our personal alignment with our heritage as evolved in Nature, we increase our chances of leading a life devoid of illness as a result of reducing the toxic burden on our body. Although I sometimes call this "my hypothesis," I am certainly not the first to propose it with respect to diet, and there are many studies available on the subject of Paleo diets [11]. However, the personal path I took to arrive at this hypothesis and the conclusions drawn from it are very different.

What I have found in the literature on the subject of our Paleo Ancestor diets, there is much disagreement. The studies I am familiar with either use modern hunter-gatherer societies as their models, or limit their studies to the late Paleo Era, after PA had learned to cook. These models yield vastly different results than the ones in this book, which takes into account the approximately 2.4 million years of our heritage that seems to have been ignored by others.

To avoid confusion, I choose to call my diet study starting point the Original Diet and, as you will see, my version is quite different from the others. While diet is certainly a necessary element in the health equation, it alone does not appear to be sufficient, which is why there is a large section of my other book, *The Wellness Project* (also repeated in my book *Nature's Detox Plan*), devoted to detoxification. Where possible, in each area of description, I have attempted to list what I consider the "purist" approach as well as some suggestions for those who prefer more leeway in what they eat. While the purist level may seem Spartan in today's world, the purpose of defining it is to establish the baseline for our species – the dividing line between Nature's 2.4 million-year experiment in evolving our species and our follow-on experiments. Without this baseline as a starting point, it is impossible to know with any degree of certainty what effect dietary experiments have had on our species. While some might consider the Original Diet an experiment, from my point of view what you are presently eating may well be the experiment, with the Original Diet representing the truly non-experimental, naturally evolved eating plan for humanity.

Each of us brings to the table a lifetime of following a different diet and lifestyle, and each of us has a different toxin profile that can drastically shape the outcome of our choices. Add to this our individual genetic and other variations and the picture gets more complicated. This is the reason for starting with a purist approach – because we don't have an owner's manual to consult, my goal is to get as close as possible to what Nature intended, in order to maximize the chances that this program will achieve positive results for you. Animal studies seem to bear this out – a particular species rarely experiments with their lifestyle unless compelled to do so by environmental changes, and even then, it is done with great caution. Humans on the other hand have the luxury (or perhaps curse) to experiment upon themselves without caution or even a plan of action. You can get up in the morning and decide to become a vegan, never once having to consider all the implications for your body, which may not be in favor of that decision at all.

Does everyone have to follow this diet plan to remain healthy? The answer is no. I am convinced that there are folks out there that are disposed to lead a perfectly healthy life for 100 years eating nothing but cake, ice cream and soda! Are you one of them? I feel confident that I am not. The problem with this view of health is that we only get the answer in hindsight, and since there is no dress rehearsal for life, I for one don't like the odds. I do not mind being a risk-taker in business, but not with my health.

Throughout the book, I will be suggesting literature and websites as reference material for specific issues that I discuss. Many of these references also contain additional information, in many cases regarding diet in general, that conflicts with what is suggested in this book. On the one hand, for those of you interested in comparing and contrasting differing viewpoints on what others consider ancestral diets, this should prove quite instructive. On the other hand, I hope you will find the reasoning put forward in these chapters sufficiently compelling to place The Original Diet at the top of your list.

On a last note, viewing The Original Diet as a change of lifestyle, I urge the reader to consider his/her priorities in life. This, of course, becomes a very esoteric and philosophical exercise that begs the question of why are we here? What is Nature's plan, if any? Reproduction is a clear goal of any living species, but beyond that, I have no answers except as applied to myself, and even those have changed over time. My personal answer is to set happiness as a major goal, which then shifts the inquiry to finding what makes you happy. As it turns out, Weston Price's statement that "life in all its fullness is mother nature obeyed" has rung true for me – I get a great deal of pleasure and satisfaction knowing I am doing the best I can to understand and follow a personal eating plan evolved by Nature. One purpose of writing this book is to introduce what has given me so much pleasure in the hope that it may do so for others.

Section Two – Eating Plans

Thou shouldst eat to live; not live to eat. Socrates

How can you tell the good stuff to eat from the bad? Getting the correct answer to this question is critical to one's health, since I believe that eating foods that are not in accord with your heritage may have the affect of adding toxins to your body at every meal. For many of us, doing that for decades can so burden our defense system that it cannot perform correctly, because either it is overworked, or it can no longer differentiate toxic cells from normal ones in our body, leading to autoimmune issues. If you are in good health, it may be safe to assume that you have made wise food choices, and therefore there is no need to make any dietary changes. In that case, you may want to read this section just as a matter of intellectual curiosity, or you may want to self-experiment with portions of the diet on an occasional basis just for fun.

Most readers of books that contain a diet plan assume, undoubtedly correctly, that the author is attempting to convince them to change their existing food choices and adopt the author's diet. I want to state at the outset that it is not my goal to convince the reader to change anything having to do with their diet or eating habits. My purpose is to define an eating plan that is a baseline, or starting point, defined by Nature, that is safe for anyone to eat, and which has the lowest levels of natural toxins. A reader's decision regarding adopting all or part of this diet should be based on their present level of health and desire to improve it, their heritage, and their interest in experimenting with new food choices.

Knowing the baseline (Original) diet, you can also make informed choices such as sticking to it only some of the time, like once a week, and seeing what happens to your health. You may choose to follow it only when you feel under the weather or are under stress (chronic stress is a toxin), the idea being to unburden your defense system from potentially toxic foods so it can deal with other issues. The diet is divided into three tiers of food choices, beginning with the baseline version, Tier One, which is the Original Diet, and ending up with Tier Three, which includes virtually all food choices. One simple way to navigate among these food choices is as a function of your present level of health. If you are healthy, you may wish to continue following your present food choices, narrowing them only in the event you are or become less than fully healthy, all the way to the Tier One diet choices. A lot of information is presented to assist you in making those food choices based on clues from Nature.

Ten different nutritionists may give you ten different answers to the question of what you should eat. As it turns out, they may all be correct, or not. You will see from the following discussion on diet that as our ancestors moved out of Africa and spread around the globe, they adapted to their local food sources (at least the winners did) and over many generations aligned their heritage with their food environment. If we could trace, with a great deal of certainty, our lineage on both sides of our family over many generations to a particular monolithic society somewhere in the world, and we knew their eating habits, it would be quite safe to assume that we could follow their ancestral diet without compromising our health. Since that approach is likely to be limited to only a small segment of the population, another approach is needed. I have taken the following direction. If we go back far enough into our past prior to our ancestors leaving their African roots, we will have in fact traced our common lineage (for all humans) to a single monolithic group in a fixed part of the world. Then, if we could determine their diet at that point in time, my hypothesis is that every one of us could safely eat it, and I would expect it to be very low in toxins. So, my first challenge was to find that very Ancient diet and assess its characteristics. Follow me!

One way to look at Nature in action, at least as it relates to us, is through the perspective of anthropology. That means taking a spin back 2.5 million years ago—about 100,000 generations—to when homo-erectus emerged on the global scene. The description of the human time line below is my personal distillation of many of the theories in the field as to what happened when. Please understand that the best one can do in this area is to piece together a very limited amount of fragmentary evidence and make educated inferences. Some additional information can be gleaned from studies of other primates, particularly chimpanzees, and modern hunter-gatherer societies.

From my point of view, the biggest human experiment of all in our dietary history was the use of fire to heat and/or cook potential sources of food. I will use the word cooking also to refer to merely heating food. There is no consensus among researchers as to when this event may have first occurred. Credible estimates range from 20,000 to about 150,000 years ago (a major variable is the time difference between the ability to make fire and its widespread use in cooking food). As we shall see, the very act of heating or cooking did not have an extreme impact on availability of our animal food sources. It just made it easier to chew and digest these foods, which may have led to a smaller jaw and dental changes, perhaps leaving room for a larger brain. However, cooking had a major impact on our plant sources of food.

Extensive research in this field yields the fact that a majority of potential plant foods available to PA are toxic to many humans when consumed raw, and hence were inedible until the development of cooking. Some other plant foods that might not have been extremely toxic were unavailable or impractical for eating, such as certain nuts in extremely hard shells, until heating burst the shells and made the food available. Because I consider cooking a human experiment and I want the Original Diet to predate such activity, the purist version of the diet will be looking at plant foods that are safely edible before cooking, whenever that occurred. As you will see, this simple criterion provides some surprising results when compared to other Paleo diet studies.

This is a good point to define "toxic" as we shall use it in the context of foods. The words "toxic" or "toxins" as used in this chapter refers to *natural* substances found in foods that produce a deleterious effect when ingested by humans. It does not refer to human-made toxins that affect food, such as pesticides, genetic modifications, growth hormones, etc., which I will refer to as contamination in this chapter. The natural toxin effect can range from a rapid lethal reaction to much more subtle effects produced only by prolonged ingestion of a given food. In order to assess toxicity, we will look at chemical analyses of food as well as our genetic cousins, the chimpanzees, to observe their food choices in an effort to find Nature's clues regarding what is safest to eat.

An assumption I have made in this study is that the "Out of Africa" theory of human evolution is correct – that is, our ancestors began in Africa and migrated from there to other parts of the world. It is still the major theory in the field, but there are alternative theories such as that our ancestors sprung up independently at various points of the globe and that not all originated from Africa.

The evolutionary theory we will be following begins with Homo erectus evolving onto the scene about 2.5 million years ago (call it 100,000 generations based on a 25-year reproductive cycle). If we assume cooking of food did not appear until somewhere approximately 125,000 years ago, although this date is quite approximate, we have been heating our food in some form only for the last 5,000 generations. So for the first 95,000 or so generations we were hunter/gatherers eating raw meat and plant foods. Cultivation (the planting and eating of grains) and domestication (the raising of cattle and eating dairy products) developed about 10,000 years ago. That's a mere 400 generations back, out of 100,000. The introduction of refined sugar occurred much later. So, what can we infer from this timeline?

In general, changes to diet require genetic or other adaptation. Looking at our food history, aside from cooking, the biggest changes occurred somewhat simultaneously 400 generations ago with the introduction of grains and dairy. Many scholars and alternative health practitioners think that 400 generations is not a long enough time for some people to adapt fully to these new food groups and, in fact, that may be a major factor for the cause of present day illnesses. We recognize, for instance, that a majority of the world's adult population is lactose intolerant, which, to me, is a clue from Nature that dairy is not a suitable food for many adult humans, the only adult species on Earth known to consume it as a regular part of their diet. We also see gluten intolerance as a common and insidious ailment, which is another clue from Nature regarding the consumption of grains, many of which are the seeds of grasses. The term gluten has many definitions, the usual one defining certain proteins found primarily in wheat, barley, and rye grains. Other grains such as rice, oats, and corn contain different glutinous proteins.

The introduction of agriculture—of grains, dairy, and refined sugars—paved the way for huge population growth, and the evolution of scattered clans and tribes to larger settlements and eventually cities, but many leading anthropologists see this development less as progress but rather as a monumental setback for humankind. UCLA's Jared Diamond, for instance, in an article entitled "The Worst Mistake in the History of the Human Race" [5] [12], asserts that recent discoveries suggest the switch from a hunting/gathering existence to one of agriculture, "supposedly our most decisive step toward a better life, was in many ways a catastrophe from which we have never recovered. With agriculture came the gross social and sexual inequality, the disease, and despotism that curse our existence." Specific to diet, he added that hunter/gatherers enjoyed a very varied diet, while the farmers that replaced them obtained most of their food from a few starchy crops. Cheap calories and poor nutrition were the result.

Diamond puts the timeline in perspective this way: "Hunter-gatherers practiced the most successful and longest-lasting lifestyle in human history. In contrast, we're still struggling with the mess into which agriculture has tumbled us, and it's unclear whether we can solve it. Suppose that an archaeologist who had visited us from outer space were trying to explain human history to his fellow spacelings. He might illustrate the results of his digs by a twenty-four hour clock on which one hour represents 100,000 years of real past time. If the history of the human race began at midnight, then we would now be almost at the end of our first day. We lived as hunter-gatherers for nearly the whole of that day, from midnight through dawn, noon, and sunset. Finally, at 11:54 p.m., we adopted agriculture" [5]. A few field and clinical studies were conducted in the early part of the 20th century to determine the effects of diet on physical degeneration in humans and cats. See the side box entitled Physical Degeneration and Dietary Change for more information. I will comment on these studies and their significance below.

The goal in the following section is to define the Original Diet that in theory was what our ancestors consumed for most of the 2.5 million years of our heritage, and before human technological intervention, beginning with fire. This would be the baseline diet that all of us have evolved to eat. The format used is to create a food-screening criteria (called the ABC Test™) that will lead to lists of fully acceptable foods and less acceptable foods. The result will be a tiered arrangement of food choices, starting with Tier One foods which represents the purist version of the diet in its most basic form. It happens to be the one I strive to follow because it contains the lowest amount of natural toxins of any fully nutritious diet, and hence has a minimal impact on the defense system. The term "Original Diet" as used in this book refers to the diet that is based on Tier One food choices. However, for many people, this purist or baseline version may seem too austere in its simplicity, so there will be a discussion of additional food choices that may be added from Tier Two and Three food categories, where each in turn is farther removed from the baseline version. The Tier One, or Original Diet, establishes the starting point upon which to build a diet for modern times, and is the one I have followed for some time. (A patent application has been filed covering certain aspects of the Original Diet.) I am now going to go into some detail reviewing the research that went into defining the Original Diet.

Physical Degeneration and Dietary Change

Two inquiring medical minds in the first half of the 20th century exhaustively explored the impact of dietary change on health and found dramatic consequences. The first was Weston A. Price, D.D.S., a Cleveland dentist, who traveled the world during the 1930s to study the causes of dental decay and physical degeneration that he saw on a daily basis in his practice. In his classic book *Nutrition and Physical Degeneration* [13], he reported finding healthy, straight teeth, freedom from decay, robust bodies, and resistance to disease, as common denominators among societies eating traditional diets. In stark contrast, he found rapid and consistent deterioration once native peoples switched to the "impoverished foods of civilization"— sugar, white flour, pasteurized milk, and convenience foods. Dental caries and deformed dental arches, resulting in crowded, crooked teeth and unattractive appearance were signs of physical degeneration, resulting from what he had suspected: nutritional deficiencies.

In a series of experiments with cats during the 1930s and 1940s, Francis M. Pottenger, Jr., M.D., a Los Angeles area physician, clearly demonstrated the power of dietary change. Working with some 900 cats over a ten-year period, he found that diets containing raw meat produced optimal health: good bone structure and density, wide palates with plenty of space for teeth, shiny fur, no parasites or disease, reproductive ease and gentleness. Keep in mind that cats are carnivores and evolved on raw meat.

Cooking the meat or substituting heat-processed milk for raw milk produced reproduction problems and physical degeneration in these cats, increasing with each generation. Vermin, parasites, skin diseases, and allergies increased precipitously and the animals gradually developed degenerative diseases seen in humans, along with adverse personality changes.

The changes Pottenger observed in cats paralleled the human degeneration that Price found among aboriginal peoples who had abandoned traditional diets. It does not require rocket science to see the clear parallel between the commercial, highly cooked, and processed food that we feed our companion animals and ourselves today, and the runaway prevalence of chronic illness besetting humans and pets. We have strayed afar from our evolutionary diet, and forced a similar disconnect on our animal friends, sometimes with disastrous results.

The significance of the research of Price and Pottenger was the inspiration for a California based nonprofit educational organization—called, appropriately The Price-Pottenger Nutrition Foundation (www.ppnf.org)— providing access to modern scientific validation of ancestral wisdom on nutrition, agriculture, and health. The organization's mission is to advance the quality of life through the study, application, research, and dissemination of nutritional and environmental information that can affect health in today's high-tech world.

Chapter 4 - The Tier One Original Diet

As a starting point, there is general agreement among Paleo-anthropologists that raw meat and certain plants were the basic food groups for PA — a diet with about 90,000 generations of history behind it. Moving closer to the present day in the timeline, added foods become more problematic for some people to eat without some sort of adverse health consequence, such as fish, fowl (it is not clear at what point we domesticated fowl and obtained easy access to eggs), grains, dairy, some cooked plant foods, extracted vegetable oils, and sugars. As we waltz our way through the world of food, keep in mind the "big eight" food categories, as they are affectionately called by allergists, that account for over 90% of the food allergies in the U.S. and tend to be in the top 10 worldwide. They are milk, eggs, peanuts, tree nuts, fish, shellfish, soy, and wheat. Chicken is also high on the list. As you will see, none of these foods formed a part of our Ancestor's original diet. Could this be another clue from MA? In the food group discussions, I will comment on the modern availability of some of the foods, and end with speculation on the relative proportions of each that may have been consumed.

The ABC Test

In my research to deduce Nature's baseline when it came to food, I used the anthropological record to create what I call an "ABC Test," described in the accompanying side box entitled The ABC Test for Food.

The ABC Test for Food ™

Here is how I apply the <u>A</u>vailable <u>B</u>efore <u>C</u>ivilization Test:

<u>Available</u> is somewhat tricky. By this I mean the following:

1) that the food was native to Africa, preferably tropical East Africa, considered the birthplace of our ancestors, and was preferably reachable by a barefoot human; and

2) that no human processing, including heating or cooking, was needed to either gain access to, or digest or derive nutrition from the food in its natural form; and

3) that the food is not toxic if consumed raw.

<u>Before Civilization</u> means that the food is not newly hybridized or genetically modified, but is as close as possible to the version that would be available pre-cultivation/domestication and precooking (say more than 125,000 years ago).

The acronym stands for: was the food <u>A</u>vailable <u>B</u>efore <u>C</u>ivilization? I have used this simple yardstick to determine whether a particular food or food family is likely to be one to which our ancestors naturally adapted, and thus is eligible for inclusion in the Original Diet. It has helped guide me in my efforts to make educated decisions on defining the baseline foods to eat, and even lifestyle choices to follow. It's certainly not an infallible guide, but it has worked very well for me.

In my search for Tier One foods, I looked first at where humanity originated in order to find foods common to the heritage of all humans. We know it began in Africa (probably tropical East Africa), so there was one obvious criterion for availability. Is (or was) a particular food or family of foods native to this area? If it is a fruit or vegetable, did it grow in Africa, and if it is a source of meat, did it roam in African climates? If not, the odds are it may not have been an early source of food for humans. Another criterion for the ABC test is how physically easily the food would have been to obtain. Plant foods would also have had to be non-toxic when eaten raw.

An important point of the ABC test that I want to emphasize is that of territory. Although PA began emigration from Africa over a long period of time during the Paleo era, perhaps many hundreds of thousands of years ago, for purposes of our diet discussion, we will initially confine the area of interest to tropical Africa on the presumption that the bulk of our heritage took part in this area of the world. As you will see, this limitation leads to very different conclusions as to food availability, particularly when compared to other Paleo-type diets based on modern hunter-gatherer groups spread around the world. Let's now take a closer look at each of the food categories.

Animal Foods

In hunter/gatherer societies, the hunter group did their best to find and kill or scavenge what they could with no tools or limited tools. There is speculation that PA was able to stampede herds over cliffs or into canyons even before any tools other than rocks were available. We presume that virtually all edible parts of the animal were ingested, including glands, organs, brains, blood, bone marrow, and the animal's raw intestinal contents, comprising partially digested fermented food, beneficial bacteria, and digestive enzymes. What we do not know is the amounts of the various parts consumed. For example, some carnivorous animals prefer the organs, glands, and fatty parts of their kill to the muscle meat, much of which is left for scavengers.

By examining our present dental and jaw structure, it becomes clear that we are not presently adapted to tear raw meat very efficiently, leading to the assumption of our having adapted to cooked meat. The following are some candidates for sources of animal protein and fat. All meet the ABC test, and in particular could have been eaten raw and without processing, although I personally prefer gently cooking my animal foods.

Cattle are members of the family Bovidae, which include several breeds that are native to Africa. Unfortunately, much of the beef produced in the U.S. is from cattle that are grain fed (mostly corn) in confined quarters, and are also fed or injected with growth hormones and antibiotics. Some are actually fed animal byproducts. For purposes of this baseline, the purist approach to eating beef is to eat only meat from humanely treated organic grass-fed and finished free-range cattle that were never treated with hormones or antibiotics. They are usually labeled as grass-fed. The term Natural as applied to meat is somewhat meaningless, applies to grain fed animals, and does not guarantee anything about the way they are reared. The meat for use on the Original diet is available from some health food markets and online suppliers, and usually originates from South America, New Zealand, or small ranches in the Midwest. Cattle are tropical animals not Native to North America, and cannot survive in a winter where the grass is covered by snow. So any cattle raised in the U.S., even grass-fed, needs nutritional support during winters from stored fodder, usually hay as a mixture of dried grasses.

Raising cattle on grain distorts their fatty acid profile, (see the section on essential fatty acids below) and is not what nature intended. The health effect on humans consuming this meat is unknown. A less than purist approach might be occasionally to eat grain-fed beef, but be sure it is organic feed, and that it is hormone- and antibiotic-free, bearing in mind that eating this meat frequently could be a health-risk factor of unknown proportions. For those interested in the grain/grass-fed issues, I suggest visiting the site of the Weston A. Price Foundation [7]. This foundation evolved from the Price-Pottenger Nutrition Foundation [13], both of which are committed to promulgating the teachings of Weston Price.

Buffalo, or bison, is another option, and they also belong to the family Bovidae. American buffalo can be found that has been grass-fed, or sometimes grass-fed and grain-finished. The finishing step takes place before the animals are put on the market, and is used as a last minute effort to fatten them up to yield a higher price. The adverse effect of grain finishing on the health of a human consuming the meat is unknown, but it is likely that these effects are less than those from eating fully grain-fed buffalo. Grass-fed and finished buffalo are available from small U.S. farms and farm cooperatives, including NorthStar Bison [14]. Purist and less than purist approaches discussed above for beef also apply here. The bottom line is that the longer the animal is free-range grass-fed during its lifetime, the closer its meat composition will be to that which was intended by Nature.

Another choice is lamb, the meat of young sheep, also members of the family Bovidae. Much of the lamb on the market is from fully grass-fed sheep, and my favorite is from New Zealand. Goat and other ruminant animals can join the list. Deer, elk, caribou, and moose (from the family Cervidae) do not appear to be native to Africa, but antelope is a candidate, as is goat.

Pork is from swine of the family Suidae, some species of which are native to Africa. For example, the bush pig is a food source for chimpanzees. One of the potential issues with pork meeting the ABC test today is that eating the meat raw can lead to toxic bacterial infections such as trichinosis if the pork is not raised in a natural environment, but this would not have been an issue for PA. If pork is of interest, look for Certified Humane Pork that is hopefully also free-range and organic-fed. While there is a USDA trichinae-free certification program for pork, I am not aware of any pork producers that have implemented it.

I am including ostrich in this category since it passes the ABC test. Although a bird, ostrich is flightless and hence was much easier prey for PA, making it likely as a food source much earlier than winged birds. Ostrich meat is delicious and available from a variety of suppliers, such as Blackwing Meats [15]. The main problem I have with ostrich is its low fat content, which leaves me hungry. Interested readers can do follow-up research of other animal families using the guidelines above.

Regarding the fat content of prey animals, I have concentrated in this section on animal families that are readily accessible to Western cultures, but in fact, there are very many more animal families native to Africa that are now either endangered, extinct, or simply unavailable as food. A simple example is the hippopotamus, distantly related to the whale! If I, as a hunter-gatherer, had a choice between a lean goat or a chunky hippo for dinner, I would choose the hippo just based on the larger amount of fat present in bigger animals (not factoring in the difficulty of obtaining that dinner!).

Some Paleo diet studies have concluded that while PA would certainly have preferred the fattiest part of animals, he/she would actually have had a relatively low animal fat dietary intake. This is based on their analysis of, for example the animal fat content of caribou and its seasonal variations (higher fat content in the fall and winter). Caribou, related to reindeer, is not native to tropical Africa, and is unlikely to have been a PA food until their emigration to the Northern climates in later periods. Also, traditional seasons do not exist in the tropics of PA, where the weather is either wet or dry, but there is no fall or winter. Other Paleo diets are based on studies of modern hunter-gatherers such as the Inuit, who are certainly not representative of life in the tropical Paleo era. Thus, it is easy to come to very different "ancient" diet conclusions if these distinctions are not clearly established. Of course, it is difficult to intuit what did take place more than 10,000 years ago in tropical Africa, but that is what this section is attempting to do.

Now, let's take a look at what portions of the meat were eaten. I prefer fatty cuts of meat because of their taste and because they are very satiating. Some studies have shown that hunter-gatherers universally sought out animal fat. In many cases, it is not easy to find high-fat cuts, so I supplement my diet with additional animal fat. I use my gut feelings to tell me when I have had enough – I feel full. Our ancestors are very likely to have eaten the animal glands and other organs, and there is evidence from studies of Inuit and American Indian groups that the intestinal contents of the animals were also consumed [16]. In the case of ruminants, this would include fermented or partially fermented grasses, along with the enzymes and bacteria from the animal gut. I discuss a particular group of those bacteria called spore-formers in the dirt section below.

Many folks do not like to eat animal glands and other organs or find them difficult to obtain. Toxicity is another potential deterrent created by modern farming and ranch practices, particularly related to consuming brain and liver tissue. An unknown issue is whether glands and other organs need to be eaten raw to derive all of their nutritional benefits. As an alternative, one can take various food supplements with each meal, discussed further below. The intestinal contents of prey would be even harder to come by in today's markets, so I suggest in later sections ways of either adding some fermented foods to the diet as a substitute, or supplementing with some of the healthy spore-forming bacteria found in animal intestines. There is also evidence that our Ancestors broke apart the bones of the animals and ate the marrow, which is filled with nutrients such as gelatin. To fill this gap, you might consider obtaining marrowbones from your butcher and using them to make soup. Recipes can be found in the book *Nourishing Traditions* by Sally Fallon [17]. More information on gelatin can be found in the supplement section below.

In his travels, Weston Price found that the Masai tribe in Africa drank cow's blood as part of their diet, and reading this bit of information led me to a fascinating bit of sleuthing. I remembered drinking "beef tea" as a kid, which my mother made by boiling meat for a long time and collecting the juice, which I devoured. I vividly recall how salty it was, and visually it reminded me of blood. Well, one of the pieces of the puzzle that had been bothering me for some time was the salt content of the PA diet. Most of the Paleo diet gurus have come to the conclusion that such diets were very low in salt, which seemed incongruous with the electrolyte needs of a hunter-gatherer running around in tropical Africa, coupled the fact that MA has provided us with salt taste buds. Just ask any marathon runner how long he/she would last on a low salt diet.

So I decided to look into the salt content of blood, and the results were quite shocking. My analysis went something like this: the sodium chloride content of blood is estimated to be about 0.9%, or about 9 grams per liter, which is also the ratio used to make isotonic salt solutions for intravenous use in hospitals. Most mammals have a whole blood volume in milliliters that is about 5-7% of the weight of the animal in kilograms.

A typical cow, depending on her size, contains somewhere between 25 and 40 liters of blood, which yields between 225 and 360 grams of salt! That is an enormous amount – between a half and three quarters of a pound of salt just in the blood of a cow [18]. Imagine a hippo or a mammoth – they would be virtual salt farms.

Well, it is not rocket science for me to jump to the conclusion that PA had all the salt he/she could possibly desire, just from the blood of their prey. Salt is an important part of the Original Diet, and I discuss it more thoroughly in later sections of the book. It also turns out that many modern cultures throughout the world do consume animal blood, but tend to disguise it with names like black pudding, and other names for what is really blood sausage.

Excluded from the animal category for the Original Diet are any prepared forms of meat, such as sausages or cured meats. In the event you are interested in obtaining the acceptable animal products mentioned in this section, many of them, including glands and other organs, and bone stock are available from US Original Meats [19].

For those concerned with cholesterol, saturated fats, and heart disease, see the box entitled Cholesterol Commentary for additional insights. Here is the short form. Can saturated fat contribute to heart disease? Yes, but not for any of the reasons put forth by the medical community.

Can elevated cholesterol be a marker for heart disease? Again, yes, but not for any of the reasons put forth by the medical community. From my research, the medical community reasonings regarding saturated fat and cholesterol are examples of faulty experiments where there is no controlled baseline, where necessary and sufficient causes are mixed up, and where correlation is confused with causation. Here is how I approached these issues.

Cholesterol Commentary

I am sure the reader is aware of the saturated fat/cholesterol/heart disease information ingrained in our culture. Even some of those favoring Paleo diets seem to shy away from the saturated animal fat issue. There are studies showing the typical fatty acid composition of various animals in an effort to try to fit a Paleo diet into the politically correct saturated fat theory. Of course, having an animal analyzed in this way does not lead to the conclusion that our ancestor's fat intake mimicked the analysis, since we do not know what and how much of each part of the animal was eaten.

The first inkling I got that the saturated fat theory needed further investigation was when I ran a self-experiment that clearly demonstrated the more saturated animal fat I ate (while following the Original Diet), the lower my total cholesterol. In fact, my entire lipid profile "improved," as this term is defined by the cardiology/pharmaceutical industry. Well, that launched me (pun intended) into an investigation of the whole saturated fat/cholesterol theory of heart disease and, as you will read, magnesium deficiency surfaced as the culprit.

I presume my dismissal of the saturated fat/cholesterol issue will not satisfy those readers concerned about heart disease and/or who have a family history of such disease. I have such a family history. On my father's side, I am the longest living male in three generations (I am 66 as I write this book) – all succumbed earlier to cardiovascular illnesses. So, here is what I did to allay my fears.

Putting on my engineering cap, my first task was to check the actual condition of my arteries. The medical community would have everyone believe that a lipid profile (cholesterol profile and triglyceride blood tests) accomplishes that task. Science and common sense say that one should not measure something indirectly if it can be easily and accurately measured directly. Actually, I don't consider a lipid profile to be a test of anything reliable when it comes to the condition of my arteries, but it may be an indication of magnesium deficiency, which is related to cardiovascular health - see the magnesium factor section below.

Direct testing of artery health took me into the world of medical testing and lo and behold, there are many non-invasive, inexpensive, and accurate tests to determine directly the condition of one's arteries. The first is the carotid ultrasound test, which takes only a few minutes and displays on a computer screen a nice picture of the large arteries leading from the heart to the brain, along with real-time blood flow color-coded for velocity. Some in the medical community say this is not good enough. What about the peripheral arteries in the lower part of the body, they ask? Okay, how about a do-it-yourself free test for that? Measure the reclining blood pressure at your arm and then at your ankle (a helper comes in handy). A reading of 90% or greater (the ratio of leg to arm) is considered a good indication of unclogged peripheral arteries. This test is sometimes referred to as an ABI test (ankle/brachial pressure index).

Still others in the medical community said that ultrasound does not reliably pick up calcium deposits in the arteries. Okay, onward to a body scan. I am not a fan of x-rays because they may cause cancer, but I make an exception for a body scan, done, say, every ten years, because the potential payoff is so great. One should opt for the latest equipment, which has the lowest x-ray levels. This test is excellent for determining an arterial calcium score (the goal is zero). Lastly, I was again taken to task because I had not gotten any information about the possibility of microvascular disease – clogging of the very small arteries throughout the body. Well, I found some anecdotal evidence showing that your friendly eye doctor can give you a clue by looking at the tiny arteries and veins in the retina, which is actually easy to do as part of a regular eye exam at no additional cost. Trained doctors can give you a valuable opinion based on their findings. Lastly, I added a stress echocardiogram to the list, although I did not feel it was necessary.

So, how did I do? When I had these tests performed, I had been on some form of the Original Diet for anywhere from 15 to 20 years, eating no grains, dairy, sugars or extracted vegetable oils. Instead, I ate lots of meat, and if still hungry, I would down up to three egg yolks per day. Of course, I also took the food supplements discussed in a later section. My carotid ultrasound results were a rousing success – wide-open arteries, excellent blood flow. The peripheral blood pressure test yielded a reading of 113% (90% or better is desirable), which shocked the technician. My body scan calcium score was zero, and the radiologist confessed that his was not that low. He cautioned me that I should not take that reading as a license to go out and eat hamburgers, which is exactly what I did (no bun, no cheese, and no sauce). The eye doctor gave me a green light at my eye exam, not only for the condition of my micro arteries, but also for my eye health in general. The stress test yielded excellent results.

I have gone to some length to cover this topic because the saturated fat/cholesterol/heart disease theory is very ingrained in our cultural psyche. I will add that my wife, who is much less of a purist than I, and who had been on the Original Diet in one form or another for several years, underwent the same tests and scored perfectly as well. While some radiology labs require a prescription to do a carotid ultrasound, several companies are now doing them quite inexpensively along with some of the other tests like the ABI, without that requirement. An example is Life Line Screening [20]. Full body scans can be somewhat expensive, but the long-term consequences of not knowing the condition of your arteries can be a lot more expensive!

I made a list of items that are *suspected* causes of cardiovascular disease, and saturated fat and cholesterol are on that list. I say suspected because it is clear from the research that you can have elevated cholesterol and eat lots of saturated fat and not have heart disease, and the reverse is also true [21] [22] [23] [24]. I then made a list of items that are *known* causes of cardiovascular disease, meaning that if this item is present, you have or will develop cardiovascular disease. There is only one item on that list – *magnesium deficiency*. Are you surprised? My guess is that many in the field of heart health would also be surprised, but they shouldn't be. There is plenty of research on the subject, and I go into more depth on it in the food supplement section below [25] [26, 27].

Once I had these two lists along with reams of data on magnesium, the likely correlation between saturated fat, cholesterol, and cardiovascular disease became clear to me. Virtually everyone on the SAD (Standard American Diet) diet is deficient in the essential mineral magnesium, obtainable from food and mineral water. This deficiency is highly correlated with every facet of cardiovascular disease, from angina, arrhythmias, clogged arteries, strokes, to sudden death. Well, it just so happens that saturated fat binds with magnesium in the gut, forming compounds that reduce assimilation of the mineral. So, if you are already deficient in magnesium and increase your saturated fat intake, you will become more deficient, further increasing your chances of heart disease.

Is the solution to reduce saturated fat intake? Of course not. The solution is to cure the magnesium deficiency.

What about cholesterol? Well, magnesium deficiency can cause elevated cholesterol in some people, so a high cholesterol level can be a marker of magnesium deficiency, not a direct cause of heart disease. In fact, magnesium lowers cholesterol in the same way as statin drugs, but without the side effects [28]. It is well known that cholesterol is a necessary element to life itself – without an adequate amount, we would be sick indeed, if not dead.

Cholesterol elevation can be caused by many factors. When it is an indicator of magnesium deficiency, it is at most an indirect and unreliable marker for the real cause of heart disease, and that is what we see from the research. There are an enormous number of people with supposedly elevated cholesterol levels (say above 200 mg/dl) that do not develop heart disease. There are likewise an enormous number of people with levels below 200 mg/dl that do. In fact, the largest study of its kind, the famous Framingham Study, produced results showing that those with total cholesterol below 200 mg/dl had a higher incidence of heart disease than those with levels above 200 mg/dl. If you read some of the references I listed above on cholesterol, you will find from an analysis of the major studies on the subject that the cholesterol levels which *minimize* mortality from all causes are as follows: total cholesterol in the range of 220-280 mg/dl, and LDL levels around 150 mg/dl!

My position regarding the prevention of heart disease is to have a sufficient magnesium level in your body. Saturated fat and cholesterol are merely warning lights for the real problem. Magnesium will reappear throughout this book as one of our mineral champions.

A discussion of animal products would not be complete without some mention of insects, which are a part of the chimpanzee and many modern hunter-gatherer diets. PA would certainly have consumed them in small quantities in eating fruit.

Plant Foods

Unlike animal foods, plant foods present a variety of difficult issues relating to human diet that have been the subject of much debate in the scientific community. Remarkably, the majority of research on components of Paleo diets has been conducted for animal products, with virtually nothing on plant availability during this time period. I funded research by graduate students in the Department of Ecology, Evolution, and Marine Biology at the University of California, Santa Barbara to assist me in uncovering whatever data was available in this area, which is not very much.

As you will see, this is one major area where clues from Nature become paramount in discerning what comprise acceptable plant foods for the Original Diet. Here is the generally accepted theory, which makes great sense to me. Unlike animals that can move, run, and hide from predators to increase their chances of survival, plants are immobile. Thus, in an evolutionary sense, they were under continuous pressure to solve their survival problems by chemical means. They produce what are called secondary compounds or substances that do not contribute to their metabolism, but are designed to repel or discourage predators, ranging from other invading plants, to insects, to animals including humans [29] [30]. Basically, this is a part of the plant's defense system.

Many of these secondary compounds are toxic in a variety of ways, some of which we have yet to uncover. The ones that produce relatively immediate signs of toxicity, such as vomiting or rashes, are easy to spot. Others are much more subtle and represent a challenge to the medical community. One reason is the long period of time that may have elapsed before symptoms of toxicity become evident. These toxic substances cover a wide range of chemical compounds that produce toxic effects in very different ways. They include enzyme inhibitors, physiological irritants, allergens, and hormone disrupters. Within each of these categories are a vast number of compounds distributed throughout the plant community, and I feel confident there are many more yet to be discovered [31]. Interestingly, several insect, bird, and animal species have adapted to a few of these plant toxins and developed a synergistic relationship with specific plants that would otherwise be toxic, and I discuss this more thoroughly in the probiotics section below. There is no room in this book to delve into all of Nature's protective plant mechanisms and the wide range of ill effects they can cause on humans, and there are many books on the subject. However, I want to emphasize the importance of this clue from Nature because I believe that ignoring it has been a contributor to illness today.

When I became aware of this toxic plant issue and researched it more thoroughly, a fascinating pattern became clear. First, not all plants contain toxins, or only contain them for a portion of their growth cycle. Many fruits fall into this category, and the Darwinian rationale is as follows. The fruits with the lowest or no toxicity seem to be those that have a sweet fleshy layer covering seeds within. One objective in plant reproduction is to disseminate seeds at a distance from the parent, to increase chances of survival and reduce the competition for nutrients that would occur if a plant simply dropped its seeds. One of Nature's plans for dissemination (there are many including wind, sticking to animal hides, etc.) appears to be to package these seeds (themselves indigestible raw) in an attractive sweet outer layer to *attract* animals to consume them. The seeds pass through the intestinal tract undigested and are returned to earth along with fecal matter (a great fertilizer) some distance from the parent plant. Voila! The reproductive cycle is completed.

This is the positive side of the Darwinian analysis (plant foods naturally designed *to be* eaten), and it contains a valuable hint. Note that the seeds of the fruit are designed not to be digested, and for insurance they contain relatively strong hulls that survive gastric juices. As it turns out, if the seeds were eaten in the sense of biting through the shells, they could lead to health problems for the eater because they contain some of the toxins I referred to above. Some of these seeds can be in the form of what we call nuts or pits or stones. Just to give you some idea of the kinds of seed toxins we are talking about, does cyanide get your attention? It is in the seeds of such fruit as apples, cherries, peaches, and apricots. Swallowing these seeds raw is no problem (except for the size of some pits!) because the outer hull protects the user from the toxins.

To complete the picture for fruits, Nature has gone one step further to increase the chances of successful plant reproduction. The sweet outer shell ripens at about the same rate that the seeds inside are developing toward the point of supporting germination, so the ideal time for consumption from the plant's perspective is when the fruit is ripe. This also coincides with the point where the fruit becomes sweet. If consumed too early in an unripe state, the fruit is bitter and may be toxic at this stage.

Two of our five groups of taste buds are designed to sense sweet and bitter tastes. Is this coincidence? More likely, it is yet another clue from Nature to avoid eating bitter-tasting fruit. This is particularly true for berries, some of which are toxic. From my research, these toxic berries are universally bitter in taste, and are Nature's clue to stay away.

An attempt to compile a list of typical fruits that meet the ABC test turned out to be quite a frustrating experience. Determining what fruits are or were native to tropical East Africa, as opposed to those that were introduced later, was the first hurdle. It turns out that most of this knowledge is lost. The next problem, from what I could glean of native fruits, was to find something equivalent that could be readily obtained in Western markets. This was a problem because most of these fruits simply are not harvested to any degree anywhere (having been replaced by the fruits with which we are now familiar). The bottom line is that the list is embarrassingly short, prompting me to propose a compromise to the ABC test for this food category, which is discussed below. Keep in mind that all of the fruits you eat should be organically grown to minimize human-made chemical contamination.

The National Academies Press has published a reference that has been in the making for several years. Entitled *Lost Crops of Africa, Volume III, Fruits*, it is a summary of a limited number of both wild and cultivated fruits of Africa, with much background information [32]. The list of fruits chosen for review was biased toward those that could have a material impact on the African economy, but it is nevertheless of great interest and contains information that was not previously publicly available. An additional research aid was the reference *Edible Wild Plants of Sub-Saharan Africa* by Peters, et al. [33] Here is a summary of those fruits for which I was able to find a related fruit somewhat widely available.

Custard Apples, related to the fruit called cherimoya. Ebony, related to persimmon. Gingerbread Plums and Carissa appear to be similar to conventional plums. Imbe is related to mangosteen, sometimes referred to as the world's most delicious fruit. Medlars are related to the noni berry. Monkey Orange tastes like orange, banana, and apricot. Star Apples, which look like plums, are available in some specialty markets, as are tamarinds and sugarplums, which look like giant purple grapes. Balanites resemble dates, and butterfruit is said to resemble the mango. Many melons are on the list, including watermelon, honeydew, cantaloupe, and others.

Figs, from the Ficus genus of trees, pass the ABC test. I prefer fresh figs as opposed to dried, which are quite high in concentrated sugars. Fresh figs also appear to be a favorite chimp food. Watermelon, mentioned above, has a water content that is so high it is used as a source of drinking water during droughts in Africa. The fruit has a diuretic effect, which can act as an excellent kidney cleanse. I have found that the more congested the kidneys, the stronger the diuretic effect. Persimmons, also mentioned above, should not be eaten unripe, since they can form an obstruction in the stomach. In addition, I avoid any that are bitter or very astringent. Use your taste buds – if it is not sweet or it is very astringent (usually due to excessive tannins), do not eat it. Jujubes pass the ABC test, but are not easy to find. Let's summarize for a moment: we are looking for ripe, sweet, non-astringent, non-bitter organically-grown fruit with seeds.

We are now going to assess the possibility of broadening the fruit category beyond the few choices resulting from the ABC test. Because eating fruit seems to be in the best interest of the plants and is in keeping with Nature's plan (as evidenced by the very low toxin profiles of all sweet fruit), I am encouraged to expand our horizons in this arena without fear of compromising health. One simple variation of the ABC test is to open up the territory from Africa to the nearest area of emigration, the Middle East. As it turns out, this change adds a lot more choices in this category. Fresh dates from date palms become available. While some ripe dates fall to the ground, others require climbing skills, and for those who have visited tropical climates, it becomes obvious that even small children easily acquire such skills. Eat dates fresh, not dried, which overly concentrates the sugar. Next is citrus, including grapefruit, orange, lemon, and lime. Remember not to deliberately eat (bite) large quantities of the seeds (swallowing them whole is okay) or any bitter parts such as the rind. I tend to avoid juicing for the reasons discussed below. If the fruit has a thin skin as opposed to a thick rind, and it is not bitter, it could be eaten.

If the assumption is correct that MA wants us to eat her sweet fruit wherever it is grown, then the fruit category can be further opened up to include virtually all of the popular sweet fruits with which we are familiar, including sweet berries like raspberries and blackberries (bitter berries can be toxic). Many people love fruits because of their sweetness, which of course is Nature's plan, and it is actually fun to discover and use our sweet and bitter taste buds. I make sure all fruit is ripe before eating and I prefer those that contain seeds or a pit, as MA intended.

Tropical fruits are likely to have been in PA's diet the longest, so you may wish to choose those first. In particular, pineapple is high in enzymes useful in the digestion of protein, and I discuss this more fully in the digestive rehabilitation section below. Papaya is also high in enzyme activity but, unfortunately, a significant portion of the papaya now grown is a genetically modified variety to provide immunity to the ringspot virus and the results of such genetic manipulation on humans is unknown. I avoid any genetically modified foods, and it concerns me greatly that this activity has begun with respect to fruits.

Most of the commercially grown fruit, even organic, contain human-made contaminants on the surface, so a cleaning step is a good idea before cutting or eating. Soaking for long periods is not a good idea because this could leech out important nutrients. Using toxic chemicals to clean fruits, such as chlorine, is also counterproductive. The method I prefer is scrubbing with clean water having a few drops of iodine in it. Where possible, use glass containers in the cleaning process.

I am not a fan of juicing fruits for several reasons. First, the very act of juicing heats the fruit to a temperature that is dependent on the construction of the juicer and the speed of juicing, but in any case, this heating effect may destroy valuable nutrients including vitamins and enzymes. Further, in most juicers, the pulp is discarded, which contains very valuable parts of the fruit, not the least of which is fiber. Therefore, what is left is something akin to sugar water. Finally, juicing can crush the seeds, allowing their toxins to be released. There are many juice bars serving this sugar water under the guise of a healthy drink, but I think not. If you ate all of the whole fruit that goes into these drinks, you would surely get the runs or a serious stomachache. To add further to the injury, pre-bottled fruit juices are practically all pasteurized (sometimes disguised as "flash" pasteurized), which definitely destroys valuable nutrients. I prefer eating the fruit as MA intended – raw, whole, sweet, and ripe.

Nature's clues relating to fruit consumption provide valuable pointers for our next investigation into the other, or negative side of the Darwinian analysis (plant foods naturally designed *not to be* eaten). From the above, it seems obvious that, as part of their defense system, plants have developed methods of deterring activities that interfere with or detract from their successful reproduction. Since there is substantially more plant life than animal life on our planet, these methods are clearly effective. I want to state at the outset that this animal/plant tension has played out over millions of years and continues to do so in a very clever, very adaptive, and very complicated manner. From my research, for other than fruit, it appears that the goal of MA is to allow certain animals to eat certain parts of certain plants in certain amounts. This is a careful balancing act so that (barring human intervention) plant species do not become extinct because of animal/insect predator activity, and animals do not become extinct for lack of plant foods. If this sounds complicated it is, and I will try to provide several examples to show how some of it works.

Let's start with an investigation of how potentially edible plants reproduce, starting with the plant itself. Anything done to outright kill the plant, like uprooting it, is certainly detrimental to its reproduction. Here, we are talking about foods in the form of roots and tubers, which grow underground and require plant destruction (yanking the plant out of the ground or eating it from underneath) to obtain them. A tuber is a thickened part of the plant that is located at or below the soil line and is used by the plant to store nutrients to further its propagation. A potato is one example. Well, if our Darwinian model is correct, roots and tubers would contain some nasty stuff for most animals, including humans.

Wait a minute, you say, everybody knows that rabbits devour carrot roots, and so do humans, clearly killing the carrot plant. However, what you see in a modern garden or farm is far from what nature intended. If we take a closer look at carrots, we find out that the ancestor of our cultivated carrot is the wild carrot plant (also called Queen Anne's Lace). As found in nature, it contains carotatoxin (also referred to as falcarinol), a neurotoxin related to hemlock. As many rabbit lovers know, this plant will sicken or kill a rabbit, so, unbelievably, rabbits do not naturally eat carrots in the wild. Somewhere in the last few thousand years, humans selectively bred the raw carrot to minimize the levels of these toxins, resulting in the modern carrot, which rabbits and humans do eat.   The potential problem with this is that even the modern carrot contains some amount of these toxins, which appear to have anti-cancer properties at one dose, and are neurotoxic at another dose.   There is virtually no research on these issues, and I have no idea who, if anyone, is watching the store when it comes to the natural toxin levels in ordinary carrots.   I do not know of anyone exhibiting immediate symptoms of toxicity from eating carrots, and I feel confident that many of us have a defense system that can easily deal with it.   The point I want to make is that eating a plant part that MA did not intend to be eaten requires that our defense system deal with natural toxins, leaving less capacity for it to deal with all of the other human-made toxins that we are subjected to in our modern lifestyle, and thus increasing the chances of illness.

Yams and potatoes are also toxic if eaten raw.   In particular, potatoes, in the nightshade family, native to South America and first cultivated about 5000 years ago, contain solanine and chaconine, poisons capable of killing animals and people, and these toxins are not eliminated by cooking [34].   Like carrots, potatoes were and are specially bred by humans to ensure toxin content is below some established threshold of acceptable toxicity [35] [36] [37].   As a result of the seriousness of these toxins, there is a monitoring program in place by the USDA to check different varieties for toxin levels, based on levels that have been chosen somewhat arbitrarily as safe.   MA has really outdone herself when it comes to protecting potatoes from predators.   Even when the potato is out of the ground, exposing it to light or even bruising it can increase its toxin concentration.

Sure, zillions of potatoes have been eaten over the years with few deaths.   All potatoes contain these toxins, and the real question, which has no answer, is: what is the long-term effect of eating potatoes on a regular basis?   Clearly, our defense system is responsible for handling the toxin load, potentially reducing our immunity to more serious toxins, many of which are described in detail in the detox section of *The Wellness Project*. It is interesting that anthropology studies show that if our ancestors were to eat a raw potato, they probably also ate clay to assist in detoxification [38].   As you will see shortly, clay plays an important role in the Original Diet.   The nightshade family also includes tomatoes (native to South America), eggplant (native to India), and chili peppers (native to the

Americas).   To some extent, they all share the toxin heritage of the nightshade family.   We could go on and on regarding roots, tubers, and toxins, but I presume you get the picture.   I tend to avoid these plant parts as nutritionally unnecessary in the Original Diet, and a toxic burden on my defense system.   Let's move on to seeds.

Another way to interfere with plant reproduction is to destroy the seeds of those plants that reproduce from seeds.   As was stated earlier, seeds can take the form of nuts, as well as beans and peas.   From a review of the literature, raw seeds, beans, and peas contain a wide range of compounds toxic to humans including protease inhibitors, lectins, glucosinolates and other goitrogens, cyanogens, saponins, gossypol pigments, lathyrogens, carcinogens, and other hormone disruptors.   The range of illnesses that can be caused by these toxins extends from a stomachache to neurological damage, cardiovascular damage, hormonal issues of all kinds, and nutrient deficiencies that can lead to many illnesses, and even death.   In fact, virtually all pharmaceuticals began their life as a plant toxin, from aspirin to statin drugs.   Plant toxins can have an upside if the plan is to kill or disable something in your body in the hope that it will cure some ailment without killing or disabling you, which is how drugs work.

About 80% of the world's present human population lives on a diet based on plant seeds, roots and tubers, so how did we get here?   Enter technology in the form of fire.   It is well accepted in the nutrition community that when humans learned to cook plants, this *supposedly* either destroyed or rendered harmless the toxins they contain.   Add to this the additional technologies of seed milling, fermenting, sprouting, soaking, and plant cultivation in general, and we now have a world dependant on those portions of plants that it would seem Nature would prefer we did not eat.

This is one of the biggest nutritional experiments in the history of humanity, and has been going on since fire was used for cooking (say 5,000 generations ago), but really took off about 400 generations ago with the cultivation of grains (grass seeds).   In my opinion, for a portion of the population, it has been a faulty experiment potentially leading to illness. Of course, one could argue that except for having access to these plant foods, a substantial portion of our world population would not have sufficient food. That argument raises ethical, philosophical, and global ecological issues way beyond the scope of this book, the purpose of which is to investigate ways of maintaining the health of those of us who are fortunate to have a wide range of choices for the foods we eat. The reason the experiment of eating grains, tubers and other plant parts may lead to illness is that heating, milling, fermenting, sprouting, and soaking do not always destroy or render harmless the toxins in these foods. In some cases, such as with fermentation, this process may even *increase* the concentration of plant toxins, and we have yet to accurately identify or measure them all. Couple this with the fact that, for some of us, our heritage did not prepare our defense system to handle these toxins on a daily basis, and you have the potential for illness. The bottom line here is that we have employed technology to fool with MA by trying to defeat her plant safeguards, creating the illusion that everyone can eat foods, without any adverse consequences, that many of us are not evolutionarily designed to eat.

A classical example is wheat, made from grass seed. A growing portion of our population is being identified as intolerant of the gluten in wheat, rye and barley. Proteins in wheat can cause an autoimmune intestinal disorder in individuals who are susceptible, causing damage to the mucosal surface of the small intestine by a toxic reaction to the ingestion of gluten, which interferes with the absorption of nutrients. Attempts have been made to eliminate the gluten by sprouting or fermenting, but to no avail. Of course, other grains, even if gluten free, all derive from seeds and hence contain cocktails of other toxins in keeping with Nature's plan.

Nuts and beans are another example. Soaking supposedly renders harmless some of the toxins in these foods, such as phytates, which interfere with mineral absorption in the body, but tests show that phytates are not completely eliminated by this means, and in fact may only be reduced by a small amount. Cooking does not do the job either.

Brassica is a genus of plants in the mustard family that includes cabbage, broccoli, cauliflower, Brussels sprouts, turnips, and radishes. Their seeds include mustard and rapeseed, the source of canola oil. While none of these are native to Africa, it is instructive to see Nature in action in the composition of these "healthful" plants. Broccoli and cauliflower, known as cruciferous vegetables, are the unopened flowers and stems of the plant before it has had a chance to bloom. Removal of these parts of the plant prevents or delays reproduction, so let's see what Nature has in store for those who partake. Virtually all of these vegetables are classified as goitrogens, meaning they contain compounds that interfere with the production of thyroid hormones, primarily the uptake of iodine, which could lead to goiter and hypothyroidism, among many other problems.

The amount of animal research in this area is really enormous, reporting somewhat devastating effects of Brassica family vegetables on the thyroid health of animals. I discuss the importance of iodine in some detail in the halogen problem section of *The Wellness Project*, and show why (in particular in today's toxic environment), anything interfering with its uptake is a very bad idea. As you will see in that section, iodine is critical to the health of the entire body, not just the thyroid. It is particularly critical for maintaining breast and ovarian health in women. Considering the near epidemic proportions of thyroid conditions, particularly in women, which include hypothyroidism and Hashimoto's disease, I predict that cruciferous and other goitrogenic vegetable consumption will be found in the future to be a leading cause of many of these problems.

An excellent report on the negative and positive health characteristics of cruciferous vegetables is *Bearers of the Cross: Crucifers in the Context of Traditional Diets and Modern Science* by Chris Masterjohn, published in Wise Traditions by the Weston A. Price Foundation, Summer 2007, pp. 34-45 [7]. Steaming these vegetables reduces the goitrogens somewhat, boiling reduces them even more, but fermentation appears to increase the goitrogenic effect, leading to a potential problem with products such as sauerkraut. Raw cabbage and radishes can be as potent as prescription anti-thyroid drugs in shutting down the thyroid. Of course, we have all heard about the anti-cancer properties of cruciferous vegetables, which seem to be connected with phytonutrients, sometimes more accurately called phytochemicals (phyto means plant). Actually, the bulk of the phytonutrients du jour, such as carotenoids, anthocyanins, and resveratrol, are primarily found in fruit.

In the cruciferous group, the phytochemicals proffered are the very ones identified as toxins that interfere with or disable natural human processes. How can we reconcile this? Well, I think all we have to do is wait, and eventually MA's message to leave her plants alone will be heard. Here is just one example. The nutritional gurus isolated from these vegetables a compound called indole-3-carbinol (I3C), which was hailed as a breakthrough in breast cancer prevention, and women were taking it by the handful as a testament to the power of broccoli, so for a while it looked like nutritionists=1 and MA=0. Uh-Oh. A study in rats has shown increased colon tumors in chemically treated rats given I3C as a dietary supplement [39]. It turns out that some nasty stuff resembling dioxin (a poison) is produced by I3C, which causes DNA damage and can lead to mutations and cancer [40]. Well, at this point the score is MA=1, nutritionists =0. Not to be outdone, the nutritionists then came up with diindolyl-methane (DIM), which is formed from I3C, but you would have to eat a boatload of vegetables to get a good dose, so they have conveniently made up potent doses of the stuff. As they say in the legal biz, the jury is still out, but I am betting on MA. I am personally confident that following Nature's blueprint has all of the anti-cancer properties I need. I would also like to predict that at some time in the future, it will be obvious that, for some people, eating plants that MA does not want to be eaten is equivalent to undergoing chemotherapy at every meal, with all of the dangers, side effects, and occasional benefits connected therewith.

What about leaf vegetables? Eating a major portion of a plant leaf can destroy or interfere with plant propagation, especially if it is a small plant. The list of toxic leaf vegetables is quite long, including such innocents as spinach and wild lettuce. There are probably non-toxic leaf vegetables out there, but I for one do not feel comfortable guessing which ones are in this category. Chimps eat leaves, but unlike humans, their large hindguts are designed to digest very high fiber plants that we cannot, and perhaps this difference in anatomy also aids chimps in detoxifying some plant species that we cannot, but all of this is speculation.

How about eating sprouts? Sprouting is sometimes touted as a healthy way of eating seeds, but in fact, many sprouts have the potential of being quite toxic when eaten raw, not surprising since this is a very delicate point in the reproductive cycle of a plant. Kidney bean sprouts, buckwheat sprouts and alfalfa sprouts are some examples. I could go on and on as to attempts that have been made to remove known plant toxins from food, but the results are quite poor. Compound that with the fact that we have yet to *identify* many of the toxins in these foods and we do not know what the safe levels of ingestion are for humans over the long term, and you get the picture that we really don't know what we are doing in this area. So, for the Tier One Original Diet, designed to closely follow Nature's clues, we will not fool with her plan and, thus, we leave out seeds, nuts, beans, peas, roots, tubers, and flowers.

This decision did not come lightly. After all, this is a significant portion of the vegetable category of plant foods. So, I decided to do some "sanity checks," as follows. First, I scoured the literature to see if anyone had reached a similar conclusion for the pre-cooking human diet. In "Toxic Substances in Plants and the Food Habits of Early Man." Science 176: p.513, the authors concluded [29]:

> "Some archeologists have suggested that the importance of vegetable foods used by early man may have been grossly underestimated because vegetable materials would not persist in archeological remains. Recognition of the widespread occurrence of toxic substances might make the opposite argument more tenable; if one makes comparisons with present-day hunter-gatherer tribes, all of which possess cooking skills, the importance of vegetable foods to evolving man may have been overestimated."

This article spurred a flurry of activity in the anthropology community to address the issue of what pre-cooking hominids may have eaten, based on fossil evidence; a study of plants indigenous to tropical East Africa; and further investigation into the diets of other primates, including chimpanzees and baboons [29-31, 41-45]. There is much disagreement as to what constitutes the plant portion of a pre-fire hominid diet, but some interesting findings are that fruit was for the most part the largest category of plant food consumed by PA, with leaves and shoots supposedly a close second, very similar to the chimpanzee diet. Nuts and seeds are also on the list (chimps can use rocks to crack some nuts), but in smaller amounts. Most wild primates do not feed on grasses, grass seeds, or underground storage organs (tubers or roots) [46].

Next in my diligence study came a check against the current most prevalent foods for allergic reactions, listed earlier, which came up with peanuts (a bean), tree nuts, soy (a bean), and wheat (a seed), which would indicate late evolutionary adoption by our ancestors, leaving less time for adaptation. All in all, when factoring in what appears to be MA's plan for her plants, I am comfortable with my decision as it applies to the Tier One Original Diet.

So, who does eat plants? Herbivores, many of which are ruminant animals, meaning they have multi-chambered stomachs and a very involved digestive system evolutionarily evolved for the express purpose of eating plant material such as grass. These animals, left to their natural environment (un-tampered with by humans), have learned which plants and which parts of each plant to eat and which to avoid to maximize their survival (if only we were that smart). This takes us full circle in MA's plan, because these are the very animals we eat to maximize *our* survival. Another way to answer the question of who eats plants is that *we* do, but the animals we eat first process them, and thus we indirectly derive nutritional benefit from plants in this manner. Ah, but this is only part of the answer to who eats plants. Insects eat plants and appear to possess unique detoxification systems to deal with plant toxins. As discussed above, insects may prove to be a big missing link in our diets and another way for us to partake of plants indirectly as food.

Before leaving this plant discussion for the moment (it is continued in the section of Tier Three foods), you may well raise the question that if MA's plan is to protect the survival of species, what possible protection can be afforded to, say, buffalo, by having them hunted and killed? Here is my personal theory as to how it works, trying to second-guess MA with the help of Darwin. When animals are chased and killed, by either humans or other animals, the ones most likely to be caught are the old and infirmed who are probably beyond reproductive age, and thus have already contributed offspring to the continuance of the species. It is also likely that the overall genetic pool of the species is strengthened in general by culling those that are not the fittest, which are the ones that are easy to catch. So even if some easy to catch animals are of reproductive age, they are likely to be genetically weaker and their lineage will be eliminated, leading to stronger offspring of others that are harder to catch, improving the overall survival of the species. Perhaps this may be considered cruel in a human frame of reference, but it is obviously effective.

Water

Water is an essential part of the diet, and the kind to drink is fresh high-mineral water as found in Nature, such as spring water and the water naturally found in fruit. There is very little information available regarding PA and water, so I will have to make some hopefully educated guesses. In the tropics during the rainy season, rainwater would have collected in virtually every depression, including tree trunks and rocks, as well as in flowing streams. This water would have absorbed a high concentration of dissolved solids, particularly when found in rock pools and mountain streams, and would thus have provided an important source of minerals to the diet, such as calcium and magnesium. It would also have contained organic acids such as fulvic and humic acids, and certain healthy bacteria, all discussed in detail in the next section. I avoid highly carbonated water, as it is rarely found in natural form. As far as water containers go, cupped hands, folded leaves (chimps use this), and hollowed out plant parts, such as a watermelon shell, might have been used. Considering the climate and need for a lot of physical activity while hunting/gathering, I would assume PA sweated quite a bit and needed frequent fluid replenishment. I view water as perhaps the major source of calcium and magnesium for PA.

I do not drink water chilled or iced, and preferably not any colder than spring water, and I do not ingest ice at any time. For the gut to work correctly, it needs to be close to body temperature, which is where enzymes and other reactions work best. Pouring cold water on this process is likely to disrupt digestion, leading to future health problems. Modern water containers should be made of uncolored glass or ceramic, not plastics or metals. Ideally, only limited amounts of water should be consumed during a meal because it can dilute stomach acid, among other things, which also disturbs digestion. Drinking hot liquids with a meal, such as soups (like bone broth) or non-caffeinated fruit teas, can actually help maintain gut temperature. As far as how much water to drink each day, I use urine color as a gauge, and try to maintain it a very pale yellow, almost colorless. Below is a discussion of water filters and containers.

Hard water vs. soft water

Many people do not like so-called hard water, which is what is delivered by most municipalities. It is high in calcium and magnesium, which cause a white film on surfaces, reduce the sudsing effect of soap and detergents, and leave a plaque-like "scale" on the inside of pipes and water heaters that can eventually reduce efficiency and block lines.

Consumer discontent spawned the water-softening industry, where the customer pays for a service that replaces the calcium and magnesium with a sodium or potassium salt. Potassium and sodium are needed electrolytes in the body that are plentiful in the Original Diet, but we also need the other two electrolytes, calcium and, more importantly, magnesium (see section on magnesium below). The resultant soft water is super-sudsing slimy stuff that rarely exists in nature. While my shower door might look better and my appliances work better, what about my body? My priority is to my health. While I can always clean and replace appliances, I only have one body, so the trade-off for me is a no-brainer, meaning no soft water. I regard softened water as Frankenwater and there are dozens of studies worldwide that show a strong inverse correlation between the hardness (mineral content) of water and cardiovascular disease, primarily due to a deficiency of magnesium in soft water [47] [48]. A website containing a wealth of research on the subject is www.mgwater.com [49]. I would not bathe in soft water, let alone drink it. By the way, I will be using various terms like Frankenfood to describe a food or other product that has been so messed with by human technology that, in my opinion, it is no longer something I want to put in or on my body.

Before we continue with the hard/soft water discussion, I want to clarify some terms. Hard water usually refers to water with a high content of calcium and/or magnesium, generally in the form of bicarbonates. Healthy hard water, as shown in the research, is one that contains substantial amounts of magnesium as well as calcium. As you will see later, my view of the ideal is to have a level of magnesium that is at least fifty percent of the level of calcium. These are the waters that contribute to low levels of cardiovascular disease.

Concerning water softeners, new models of dishwashers have the option for a built in water softener to which you add salt, and I have no problem with this limited use. I know of some unscrupulous soft water marketers who scare people into thinking that the minerals that clog copper pipes will also clog one's arteries and need to be removed, an absurd bit of twisted logic. Without access to the copper-pipe-clogging minerals calcium and magnesium, a person would have no bone strength and/or be dead. In my house, I go to great pains to add lots of additional minerals back into the filtered water. From a water analysis, I get close to 3 mg of calcium and 1.5 mg of magnesium per ounce of high-mineral water, making available to me about 250 mg of calcium and 125 mg of magnesium per day just from drinking water. My assumption is that the water that PA drank contained even more of these critical minerals, so mineral supplementation becomes important, and is dealt with further below. There are many laboratories available to test home water and I encourage such testing [50].

Water filters

In today's world of contaminated drinking water, various filtering techniques are in wide use to eliminate toxins, but many of them also remove important essential minerals, or otherwise add unhealthy compounds. I avoid distilled water (I don't think it exists in Nature), reverse osmosis (RO) treated water (similar to distilled), and soft water (rarely found in Nature). Virtually all of the drinking water available to us today does require filtering to eliminate toxins.

Many healthy indigenous groups have had access to spring water packed with minerals collected on the way down from mountain heights, and sterilized by ultraviolet light from the sun. I do not think it is a coincidence that some of the longest lived groups live in mountainous areas close to free-flowing streams. In modern times, the water that reaches your home usually starts its journey from a reservoir, then goes through one or more treatment plants that add toxins such as chlorine and fluorine, then perhaps travels through an aqueduct before going underground through a pipe system. The pipes may be made of iron, plastic, copper, or ceramic, and the water picks up some of the particles of these materials. Alternatively, you may be using well water, which picks up all of the groundwater toxins that have percolated into it from human-made sources.

In order to protect consumers against bacterial buildup, since 1908, municipalities have been treating with chlorine the water they sell to consumers. Unfortunately, this element is toxic not just to bacteria but to humans as well. When chlorine reacts with organic substances, it forms compounds called chloramines, which are known carcinogens. Chlorine itself is a neurotoxin and interferes with certain hormonal processes. Municipal water may also include variable trace levels of nasty substances such as runoff residuals of fertilizers, pesticides, herbicides, and fungicides, heavy metals, cysts, viruses, fungi, bacteria, industrial wastes, rocket fuel, and prescription drugs such as antibiotics and hormones.

Drinking, showering or bathing in this stuff is a good way to add toxins to the body. In a shower, the hot water opens pores and we can inhale and absorb large amounts of the bad stuff (spas, hot, tubs, and pools add to the toxin problem with their use of chlorine, bromine, and algaecides. Therefore, water filtering is a necessary part of the Original Diet, with the goal of matching the healthy characteristics of fresh mountain stream water as closely as possible.

One option is the reverse osmosis system (RO) system, commonly used in under-the-counter kitchen filters. The problem with this method is that it removes not just the bad impurities but a lot of the good stuff as well, namely minerals. Plumbers installing RO (and distillation) filters take care to be sure that the water from the filter does not run through a copper pipe to the drinking spout. The instructions for such systems, in fact, caution not to use copper (or any metal) for this purpose. That's because RO (and distilled) water will suck the copper right out of the pipe.

For those using an RO or distillation system, there are a number of re-mineralizer systems on the market that claim to add back some of the missing minerals, primarily calcium and magnesium, and they may be worth an investigation. Another approach is to take a mineral supplement along with RO or distilled water. It seems to me that an important part of the mineral content of mountain spring water comes from the rocks over and through which the water flows as it travels down to the ocean. A very common type of such rock is a form of limestone known as dolomite. It has a high concentration of calcium and magnesium carbonate in approximately a 1.7 to 1 ratio. Carbonate forms of minerals have been dismissed by the mineral supplement industry on the basis that they have a low percentage of assimilation in the human gut. If that was in fact true, all mineral waters would seem to be useless, and they are not. Calcium and magnesium in natural mineral water appear in the form of soluble bicarbonates, which are produced when the carbonate forms of the minerals, such as in dolomite, are combined with carbon dioxide in the water.

I would rather listen to MA than the supplement industry, and I use a dolomite supplement to replicate closely the mineral content of spring water. A few years ago, dolomite supplements had a bad name because some brands contained high levels of lead. I have found a source of dolomite from a supplier who indicates they derive their dolomite from deeply buried ancient mineral deposits free of toxic metals. They test their product for lead, with a limit of ten parts per billion, a very low level [51]. While there is no safe level for lead, magnesium acts to displace and replace it in the body, so the high levels of magnesium in dolomite mitigate against even these small amounts of lead as being troublesome. One dolomite tablet with each glass of water (not with meals because it can neutralize stomach acid), up to four tablets per day (a total of 630 mg of calcium and 360 mg of magnesium), would seem to restore a good part of the natural calcium and magnesium missing from RO or distilled water. I will be discussing dolomite further in the mineral section below, but I want to emphasize its importance as a completely natural compound, undoubtedly loaded with essential trace minerals. A fascinating book discussing the health benefits of dolomite was written decades ago by Jerome Rodale, a pioneer in the health field [52].

Although I am not a fan of plastic pipes, in the case of RO or distilled water systems they are definitely required. Copper toxicity is a much-overlooked contributor to health problems including rheumatoid and osteoarthritis, bone fractures, decreased libido, panic attacks, hair loss, fatigue, and childhood hyperactivity and learning disorders. These types of filtered water should not pass through any kind of metal, including metal water bottles or cooking utensils, as the water may absorb components of the metal itself. An issue I have with many RO and distiller systems is that the drinking faucet may be made of copper or brass, so the water sitting in contact with the faucet may well be leaching metals from the faucet into the water. Copper is an important mineral for health but only in very small amounts, beyond which it is toxic [53].

Unfortunately, RO and distilled water may also absorb toxins from the plastic pipes. Why is this so? As many of you recall from science class, water is the universal solvent, and acts to dissolve solids up to the point where it is fully saturated. Well, distilled and RO water contain virtually no dissolved solids, so they act very aggressively to dissolve whatever it is they are in contact with. Opposed to this is water with a high desirable mineral content, which is close to or at saturation, and hence has very little affinity for dissolving unwanted substances, like copper and plastic from pipes and containers. This is not rocket science. Which brings up stainless steel.

Most water distillation filters use a stainless steel tank (hopefully food grade) to heat and hold the water. Stainless steel is used everywhere in the food industry, from raw ingredient containers to cooking utensils to eating utensils, as well as in medical and dental instruments. Stainless steel is the name given to iron based alloys containing at least 10% chromium. I am not a metallurgist, but I took my share of metallurgy courses in college, and it is well known that all iron alloys exposed to water and oxygen will corrode, and a popular industry spec for stainless steel allows for 0.1 mm of surface corrosion per year. So-called food-grade stainless alloys include Type 304, which contains chromium, nickel, carbon, and manganese, and is known as 18/8 stainless. Type 316 has higher corrosion resistance, and further includes molybdenum. Stainless steel is also used in water heaters and water filters. Since it is virtually impossible to avoid stainless steel, my point is to raise the possibility that small amounts of iron, chromium, nickel and molybdenum may be leaching into the food and water chain, increasing the importance of having a filter that removes metals. This corrosion factor is another reason I do not use stainless steel (or any other metal) for water containers.

Here are my filter suggestions. Starting with the simplest, for drinking water I have used under-counter (and counter-top) filters made by Doulton, a British company, and sold by many distributors [54]. The main filter uses a ceramic cartridge impregnated with silver. Many other cartridges are available for specific filter requirements, such as eliminating fluoride, and the model HIP-320 is a good choice. In a way, using ceramic mimics MA's natural rock filtration system. By the way, the bibliography section and Appendix C at the end of this book contains many website references to potential sources of information and/or products.

For a shower filter, I have used the Shower Soft Filter by Hydro-Flow Filtration Systems [13], and it is easily installed in most showers just behind the showerhead. It uses KDF, a filter medium that works well in cold or hot water to remove chlorine and many organic toxins, so your shower (and you) will no longer have a chlorine odor. For those who like to take baths, the tub can be filled with water from the shower.

One of the most intriguing water filters on the market is called the Wellness Filter, a Japanese product line ranging from showerheads to whole-house systems that is designed to replicate mountain stream water [55]. The filters not only remove most of the bad stuff (fluoride is an exception), many models re-insert into the water desirable minerals mined from various volcanic mountain locations in Japan which have been studied for millennia for their healing properties. They mine the rock from those locations, pulverized it, and layer it into their filters, which also include carbon, KDF, and magnetics. Apparently, Japanese hospitals and some of their Olympic teams are using these filters, and high-end American restaurants have started to install them as well. I have a whole-house version of the filter that works well. It is programmed to backwash weekly, and no media (filter element) replacement is required for many years.

For communities that have fluoridated water, the filter problem is substantially more complicated. Eliminating fluoride requires either RO, or distillation, or a special media filter, so for those unlucky enough to be in a community that fluoridates its water, one of these filters would be useful wherever there is a drinking water spout. The media filter uses aluminum oxide, so there should be a KDF and carbon filter following it to remove any aluminum oxide that may leach into the water. The Doulton filter does the job with the right selection of filter elements. Users of the whole house Wellness filter, which does not remove fluoride, may need to include a Doulton unit at drinking stations. I do not know of any whole house system for removing fluoride, leaving one vulnerable to shower inhalation and absorption of this potentially toxic mineral.

Alternatives are to petition local government to get the fluoride out of the water (it is a nasty toxin), or to move (I moved).

Water Bottles

The plastic water bottle is everywhere, and it is difficult to pick a starting point to discuss its toxicity because the playing field is rapidly expanding.   Let's begin with the most popular plastic, polyethylene terephthalate (PET), shown as a #1 inside a triangle on the bottle bottom, and used by virtually all brands of bottled water.   A somewhat recent study showed elevated levels of the metal antimony leaching from these bottles into the water [56].   Antimony is nasty stuff, and while the amounts measured were below the supposedly acceptable level, they were hundreds of times higher than levels normally found in drinking water, not surprising since antimony trioxide is used in the production of PET. There is almost no information on the hazards of oral ingestion of antimony, but it is a cumulative metal with a long half-life, and it is rated as carcinogenic. It also appears in breast milk, crosses the placenta, and may be a cause of miscarriages. Compound this with the fact that much of the bottled water is made using the RO process, so it is in a state where it can aggressively absorb bad stuff, like antimony. Over thirty years ago, it was reported that plants watered with water stored in PET bottles did not grow as well as those watered without using plastic [57], which raises all sorts of issues as to the impact on plant foods of plastic used in irrigation systems.

Moving on to polycarbonate bottles, these are the hard plastic ones that sometimes come in colors, or have a bluish cast in a semitransparent style, with a #7 on the bottom in a triangle. They leach bisphenol-A (BPA) into the water, and this chemical, which is also found in soup and soda can liners, is an estrogen mimic that can cause hormone havoc. It had been found in baby bottles, pacifiers and other toys, and because it can be particularly devastating to children, its use has been banned in many of these products [58]. Washing these bottles with a detergent can worsen the situation. I have seen people at the market line up with their re-usable # 7 water containers and put money into a machine that generates RO water from tap water. Here again, putting mineral-free RO water into plastic is not a great idea, and I wonder if there is any real health benefit for their efforts. So far, plastic containers labeled

#2, #4 or #5 have escaped the toxic tide, but my guess would be it is only a matter of time before they too meet the fate of #1 and #7. This is not rocket science. All plastic containers are toxic.

Many health-minded people are switching to metal bottles, and stainless steel is becoming the vogue. I already covered the issues I have with stainless, and I would not drink from them or cook in metal. Other fashion bottles claim to have inert liners of one sort or another, such as epoxy. Most common epoxy resins are produced from a reaction between epichlorohydrin and bisphenol-A. We dealt with bisphenol-A above, and epichlorohydrin is a known reproductive toxin. Many epoxies are FDA approved for contact with foods, and they may be somewhat inert until scratched or otherwise abraded. Those who insist upon metal might want to consider drinking out of a sterling silver goblet (see side box below).

A Non-Toxic Plastic Water Bottle?

Many folks know of the potential toxicity of plastic water bottles, but are not willing to lug around a heavy glass one. I will be commenting further about the unique properties of silver, and certainly one could safely drink out of a silver cup. I came up with the idea of combining silver and a plastic such as polycarbonate with two objectives in mind. First is to use the silver to bind with the toxic components in the plastic to prevent them from being leached into the water. Second is to provide a source of silver ions on the inside and outside surface of the container to disinfect the water in the container, and to disinfect the hands of the user on the outside of the container, in an effort to avoid the spread of nasty bacterial infections such as MRSA (methicillin resistant staphylococcus aureus). I have filed a patent application covering the concept in the hope of attracting a company to commercialize it.

So what's left to drink out of? How about good old glass? Yes, it can break on impact, and it's a lot heavier than plastic but it's the best and safest choice, along with uncolored ceramic. Some flat mineral water products are sold in glass bottles, such as Evian, and they can be reused. Alternatively, glass bottles of all shapes and sizes can be purchased online from a variety of sources [59]. I particularly like swing-top locking flask designs. Cloth water bottle holders with straps are available to minimize the chances of breakage, and can also be used to make a fashion statement!

Dirt

By dirt, I mean soil, but the word dirt is so much more dramatic! Is dirt an acceptable food? Few people appreciate the fact that soil itself is a form of food. It is unlikely that PA washed off what she/he ate, and so ingested some soil with fruit, animal prey, and drinking water. Surprisingly, soil contains many beneficial bacteria, amino acids, and trace minerals, as well as other compounds that we have yet to identify. From my research, there appear to be four separate groups of soil materials that contribute to health both for animals (including humans), and plants.

The first group is in the form of acids named fulvic and humic acids, which are major constituents of what you may be familiar with as potting soil, humus, or peat moss. This material is the accumulation of partially decayed vegetable matter, before it turns into coal or oil. It is great for plant growth, and some interesting research has been conducted regarding the beneficial effects from human consumption [60]. What becomes clear from this research is the importance of starting with very clean soil, free of toxins. Put another way, if you ingest toxic soil, it will toxify you, which appears to have happened on at least some occasions [61]. My approach was to find suppliers who have been providing these soil components as supplements for human consumption for a decade or more. In the U.S., the predominant source of soil for these supplements is known as the Fruitland Formation, located in Northwestern New Mexico. This shale formation from which the soil is taken is the remains of an ancient shallow fresh-water sea dating from about 80 million years ago. Several companies have been mining the soil from it for decades for use as soil conditioners as well as for animal and human use [62] [63]. Some of the cited human benefits include improved mineral utilization, and antiviral properties. These soil acids also bind with heavy metals so they can pass out of the body, and act as an immune system stimulant.

One of several companies that have been offering soil products for human use for some time is Morningstar Minerals [64], who offer capsules and liquids containing high concentrations of fulvic and humic acids. The products I use are those with minimal processing, referred to as Immune Boost 77 (capsules) and Vitality Boost HA (liquid). It seems to me that PA would have ingested a daily dose of these acids by drinking water found in tree and rock depressions, and even in flowing stream water that picks up soil along the way. I add one capsule or one ounce of the liquid each day to my drinking water as a way of more closely duplicating PA's diet. Note that the high carbon content of these supplements may cause darkening of the water and the stool.

The second group of materials from soil is bacteria, and they turn out to be an important component of the Original Diet, as well as an important part of the detox protocols. These bacteria, sometimes inaccurately referred to as soil based organisms (SBOs), are quite different from the conventional probiotics most of us are familiar with, such as acidophilus, so to avoid confusion I will not refer to them as probiotics. While these organisms are certainly found in great quantity in soil, it really is not clear where they might have originated. In addition to soil, they are found throughout nature in water, dust, air, and in the intestines of animals, insects, and sea life, but they are not native to the human gut and do not take up permanent residence there, unlike conventional probiotics. They survive stomach acid, thrive in an oxygen environment, have the ability to form spores (actually endospores) and can bind with toxins.

The ability to form spores has resulted in the name *spore-formers* being used to describe these bacteria, and I will refer to them as such. I will be going into some detail in this section because I believe they are a very important missing ingredient in our diets that can have a profound positive effect on our health. Some of the reasons they are missing include the widespread use of fungicides and pesticides in the soil, and the use of disinfectants such as chlorine in our water supplies, all of which can prevent spore-formers from proliferating.

There is research being performed on spore-formers in the belief that they may eventually replace conventional antibiotics, which are rapidly becoming obsolete due to bacterial resistance. Spore-formers could have appeared in PA's diet from dirt or dust on fruit, in drinking water, and from the intestinal contents of their animal prey, discussed in the probiotics section below.

For some of my comments, I will be drawing from an excellent review of the subject entitled *The Use of Bacterial Spore Formers as*

Probiotics by H. Hong, et al. [65]. One simplified way to understand spore-forming bacteria is to use a seed analogy. Just like a plant seed that has a strong coating protecting the embryo, the spore-formers have a strong coating protecting an endospore. They can lie dormant for years until germinated by being placed in a suitable environment, which usually includes a liquid. The human gut is an ideal environment for many of these species to germinate. As we have seen, plant seeds do not find our gut hospitable for germination and, of course, they contain all of the natural toxins discussed earlier. I like to think of the spore-formers as MA's way of providing us with "friendly seeds" designed to grow for a short time in the "soil" of our intestines and provide great health benefits. Having said that, there are spore-formers that are quite nasty, such as anthrax, so it behooves us to tread with care in this area.

Although research is still in its infancy as it applies to humans, the potential benefits that can be derived from these bacteria are somewhat overwhelming. From what is known, immune system stimulation and the generation of unique antimicrobials are just two areas of great interest. A third benefit is that of competitive exclusion (CE), where the spore-formers take up temporary residence, and through a variety of poorly understood mechanisms, exclude pathogens from adhering to the gut wall. At one time, I thought that conventional probiotics could fill this role, but from my experience, they cannot hold a candle to the spore-formers in the pathogen exclusion arena. Yet another area of interest for spore-formers is that of cardiovascular disease. A fermented soy product called natto (and nattokinase) has been touted as preventing heart attacks and cancer, among other benefits. Well, natto is made by fermenting soy with bacillus subtilis, a spore-former, so it is certainly possible that it is the subtilis, not the soy, which is responsible for the benefits.

Reading between the lines of some of the research studies [66], I ponder the following. If ingesting a somewhat continuous supply of spore-formers with our food (they tend to last less than 30 days in the human gut) can effectively exclude pathogens from taking up residence, could they be a preventive for a whole host of bad guys such as salmonella, C. difficile, H. pylori, MRSA, anthrax, and the bacteria responsible for malaria and Lyme disease? In the fungal arena, there is a great deal of evidence that spore-formers can exclude Candida and other fungi from the gut. Spore-formers are also known bioinsecticides, opening up a fertile area of research into a natural form of mosquito control [67]. By now, you may be sensing a great deal of excitement on my part for the goodies described in this dirt section of the diet, and at one point I thought of naming the Original Diet "The Dirt Diet™," but well-meaning friends suggested I reserve it as an alternate title.

Here is how I use spore-formers as part of the diet. My approach, as in the case of the humic and fulvic acid products, is to find suppliers that have been providing spore-formers for human use for a decade or more. Several species of the *bacillus* genus of spore formers have seen extensive use in human supplements worldwide, and they include b. subtilis, b. licheniformis, b. megaterium, b. clausii, b. coagulans, and b. laterosporus. After some research, I have chosen two species that have a long history of non-pathogenic use and favorable symptom relief. The first is bacillus coagulans, which is also called (somewhat incorrectly) lactobacillus sporogenes. It is supplied as capsules under the lactobacillus sporogenes name by both Thorne Research [68] and Pure Encapsulations [69]. The second species is bacillus laterosporus, strain BOD [70], which is widely distributed by O'Donnell Formulas under the names Flora Balance and Latero-Flora as capsules and powder. These supplements can be purchased at many supplement retailers [71]. Because they are found in soil and water in their natural environment, I take them with drinking water along with the humic-fulvic acid supplements. For a maintenance dose, I use one capsule per day, or an equivalent dose of the powder.

Although not a normal dietary component, other very valuable forms of dirt -known as clays- have always been used in the animal kingdom and among humans as a detoxifying agent, and form the third group of materials that make up dirt. I have devoted an entire section to the health benefits of clay in the detox section of *The Wellness Project*. As you will see in that discussion, before cooking allowed PA to experiment with eating plants that are toxic when raw, if it was necessary to eat these foods or face starvation, PA sought out certain clays to eat with the food. These acted to either adsorb or otherwise detoxify the toxic compounds in the plant food. Although we avoid these naturally toxic foods in the Original Diet, we can use clay to assist in removing a variety of other toxins from our body, and as a digestive aid for those wanting to switch diets.

The fourth component of dirt for purposes of our discussion is dolomite, which was discussed in the section on water. Dolomite, a rock that is a form of limestone, is widely found on and in the Earth's surface as stone formations and as natural sediment in the soil. It is discussed further in the mineral section below.

In summary, there are four components to dirt as it is defined for the Original Diet: humic/fulvic acids, spore-forming bacteria, clay, and dolomite.

Chapter 5 - Summary of The Tier One Original Diet

This completes the analysis section defining acceptable foods for the Tier One (and purist) diet of our Paleo Ancestors, to the extent I have been able to glean information from my research. Table 2 summarizes these findings. Recall that the purpose of this diet study was to establish a baseline set of foods that most closely resembled those of our ancient pre-fire ancestors before any tampering by human technology.

Table 2
The Tier One Original Diet

Here are the general food categories for the Tier One Original Diet. Within each category, the ABC test can be applied to a specific food to get an idea of its suitability:

- Animal protein and fat, including glands and other organs, bone marrow, blood, and intestinal contents from free-range hormone/antibiotic-free animals that eat their natural diet
- Non-Bitter Ripe Fruit - organically grown
- Soil: humic/fulvic acids and spore-forming bacteria
- Mineral-rich water with a high content of magnesium

The premise is these foods most closely align with our nutritional heritage, they can be eaten by all humans without harm, and will provide nutritional support for a healthy life, as demonstrated by 90,000 past generations. I am not proposing that everyone must follow the Original Diet to remain healthy. I am proposing it as a tool for use in the field of nutrition as a standard of comparison against which other foods and diets can be compared. This is based on my conclusion that The Original Diet contains the lowest amount of natural toxins (phytates, oxalates, trypsin and other protease inhibitors, lectins, glucosinolates and other goitrogens, cyanogens, tannins, saponins, gossypol pigments, lathyrogens, carcinogens, and various other hormone disruptors) and has an enormously successful evolutionary history behind it.

In the following sections, I examine the food groups that have, so far, been excluded from Tier One. I attempt to make educated guesses as to what foods might be added, in the framework of a cost/benefit analysis as it applies to the possible detrimental effects on our health.

Before moving past the Tier One Original Diet, let's complete the discussion by looking at how much animal food vs. plant food might be consumed. One way to answer the question is to look at the potential macronutrients derived from each category versus what is generally accepted as the minimum required in a human diet. Clearly, there is very little fat or protein in fruit compared to animal products, which are low in carbohydrates. From my personal experience, the most critical macronutrient component of the Original Diet is *animal fat*. Unless there is enough fat in the diet, it will not prove satisfying, and can even lead to annoying symptoms such as fatigue and diarrhea. I am not the first to have come to this conclusion in connection with ancestral diets.

Vilhjalmur Stefansson was an anthropologist and Arctic explorer who spent many years living with the Eskimos and Indians of Northern Canada. He reported that wild male ruminants like elk and caribou carry a large slab of back fat, weighing as much as 40 to 50 pounds. The Indians and Eskimo hunted older male animals preferentially because they wanted this back-slab fat, as well as the highly saturated fat found around the kidneys. In his book *The Fat of the Land*, he wrote:

> "The groups that depend on the blubber animals are the most
> fortunate in the hunting way of life, for they never suffer from
> fat-hunger. This trouble is worst, so far as North America is
> concerned, among those forest Indians who depend at times on

rabbits, the leanest animal in the North, and who develop the extreme fat-hunger known as rabbit-starvation. Rabbit eaters, if they have no fat from another source—beaver, moose, fish—will develop diarrhea in about a week, with headache, lassitude, a vague discomfort. If there are enough rabbits, the people eat till their stomachs are distended; but no matter how much they eat they feel unsatisfied" [72].

Stefansson is unique in having taken part in a fascinating experiment in which he and a colleague undertook a physician-supervised one-year program in 1929 where they ate nothing but meat, attempting to duplicate the diet they had followed in the Arctic years earlier. The fat content was increased early in the experiment based on the participant's requests. A March 31, 1930, article in *Time* magazine reported on the experiment:

> "Last August four physicians of the Russell Sage Institute at Bellevue Hospital, New York, announced after three months deliberation that Vilhjalmur Stefansson and Karsten Anderson, Arctic explorers, had not harmed themselves by living on an all-meat diet for one year and ten days. Said the physicians: "In general, white men, after they have become accustomed to the omission of other foods from their diet, may subsist on an exclusive meat diet in a temperate climate without damage to health or efficiency." Said Meat-Eater Stefansson: "I am wide awake and am more aggressive in my work than I was before I started this test. . . .""

With the exception of cooking my meat, I personally have followed the Original Diet in one form or another for many years, while also experimenting with adding other food categories. I feel best when I stick closely to the Original Diet. The average macronutrient ratios that seem to work best for me as a somewhat sedentary researcher are one part carbohydrate to two parts protein to between three and four parts fat, by weight. For a 2,000 calorie per day diet, this yields ten to fifteen percent of calories from carbohydrates (50 to 75 grams), twenty to thirty percent of calories from protein (100 to 150 grams) and sixty to seventy percent of calories from fats (133 to 155 grams). Other experimenting with this diet may choose very different macronutrient ratios.

Most of the research in the field of pre-agriculture hominid diets centers on post-fire modern hunter-gatherer nutrient intake, which is not relevant to this study and produces very different results. One example is the Kalahari Bushmen, mostly a gatherer society, who learned to use fire to open the hard shells of mongongo nuts. The heat also probably reduces the toxin load of the nut. Our PA had no such luxury and, consequently, a dietary comparison would be somewhat meaningless. Still other research uses indigenous populations that have developed skills and tools not found in our area of interest, such as fishing and some domestication or cultivation.

I do have a personal theory, however, as to what might have taken place in PA's time, based on my experiments. Lots of studies place an optimum dietary protein content in the 20-30% range, where larger amounts can overtax the digestive system and even lead to rabbit starvation, and lower amounts are insufficient to support energy needs. That leaves 70-80% to be divided between carbs and fats. Well, I presume PA's diet was quite opportunistic, depending on the fat content of the animal prey and the availability of fruit. So, perhaps one day (or week) PA's diet might have been mostly fat if a large animal was caught, or mostly fruit and protein from small animals if not. How that averaged out is anyone's guess, but if it was me, I'd go for the fat to the extent it was available, before grabbing the fruit.

Put another way, trying to assign macronutrient ratios to PA's diet is not realistic. PA did not have the luxury of plucking foods from a supermarket, but instead took advantage of what was available. The closest we can figure is that animal protein was probably readily available, even if it had to come from small lean animals at times, so the real variables were carbs and fat. As far as how often to eat, three times per day works for me.

Using a 2000-calorie diet as an example, with a carbohydrate allowance of 50 to 75 grams, let's see how extensively we can indulge ourselves with fruit. How about this: a half grapefruit with breakfast (12 gm), a large wedge of watermelon with lunch (21 gm), and a bowl of fresh raspberries with dinner (10 gm), leaving three fresh figs (30 gm), or three passion fruit (15 gm) available with snacks (USDA database). Hardly a spartan diet.

I don't know if PA ate snacks, but here is a suggestion that works well with the Original Diet but does not strictly meet the ABC test. Pemmican is a modern food believed to have been developed by the American Indians. It consists of dried pulverized meat, animal fat, and occasionally some dried berries, and meets the ABC test if we allow for a minimal amount of processing (drying). Many recipes are available for do-it-yourselfers, using grass-fed animals for the protein and fat, and fruit as a sweetener. Plain jerky (dried meat) is another possibility, but I find it to be too low in fat, and so do not use it. Pre-made pemmican is available from some online meat suppliers such as US Original Meats, mentioned previously [19].

I have not mentioned caloric intake in the discussion of the Original Diet for a number of reasons. First, the Original Diet is not about losing weight, it is about getting and staying healthy. Second, it is difficult to overeat on this diet because of the satiating effect of animal fat. Of course, if the amount of energy your body derived from your food intake exceeds your energy expenditure, the excess will accumulate, generally as body fat. Regarding derived energy from food, if your body was a perfect energy-converting machine, in theory it could derive from food its entire caloric value, which is the maximum amount of potential energy contained in the food, sort of like the BTU (British Thermal Units) rating of automobile fuel. The energy conversion takes place in the digestive system, and requires a whole symphony of processes to be successful, which are dependent on enzyme reactions, bacterial fermentations, fat emulsification, and some we have yet to figure out.

Assuming your gut is less than perfect, which I fear is mostly the case these days, then the energy derived from food will be less that the caloric maximum, and can vary based on the type of food. For example, for those who no longer have their gall bladder, chances are they digest fats inefficiently because of a bile acid deficit (correctable by supplementation as described below). So some of those who follow the Original Diet may experience a weight loss because of the high fat content. Where does the unconverted energy go? Well, let's use a car as an example. If your car is in need of a tune-up, it will most likely not burn fuel efficiently, wasting a portion of the potential energy of the fuel, and your MPG (miles per gallon) will suffer. Where does the unburned fuel go? Look at what comes out the tailpipe. The same with people – look in the toilet bowl. Poor fat-converters often exhibit steatorrhea, or fatty foul-smelling floating stools. Chronic diarrhea or constipation can also be clues to malabsorption, where a portion of food passes through you undigested. This really is not rocket science, yet I have seen a great deal of puzzlement in the nutrition field as to how, for some people, an equal number of food calories ingested can produce different results in that person as a function of the macronutrient composition, and all kinds of exotic theories have been concocted to explain it. This mystery has even been given the name Metabolic Advantage, when in fact it is a metabolic *disadvantage*. One of the goals of The Original Diet is to get the gut into fine shape so that it can derive the maximum energy benefit from foods, regardless of the composition of your diet.

From years of studying the natural toxicity of foods, I feel comfortable saying that the Tier One Original Diet is the lowest in natural toxins, having virtually eliminated phytates, oxalates, trypsin and other protease inhibitors, lectins, glucosinolates and other goitrogens, cyanogens, tannins, saponins, gossypol pigments, lathyrogens, carcinogens, and other hormone disruptors. The chances of having a true allergic reaction to meat or fruit are close to zero. However, those who have a digestive system in disarray as a result of toxins may well experience a reaction to these foods, and this is further dealt with below. Additionally, when beginning the Original Diet after following a SAD diet, some may think they are having an allergic reaction to the new foods, but it is more likely their gut is going through shock in attempting a return to its natural state.

Some people that suffer from hypoglycemia (low blood sugar) might have a problem eating large amounts of fruit, which causes their blood sugar to dip. It has been my experience that hypoglycemia results from an endocrine system disorder, usually relating to pituitary, adrenal and/or thyroid issues, discussed in *The Wellness Project*. Until this condition can be dealt with, eating fruit along with even a small amount of animal fat and/or protein, such as some pemmican or even a few desiccated liver tablets (described below in the supplement section) should temporarily eliminate the low blood sugar problem.

Fasting has no place in the Original Diet, but for those eating any other diet, such as the SAD diet, I would certainly encourage it. Anything that decreases the intake of toxic foods is certain to improve health, which is probably why some folks eating the wrong foods report that they feel better when they fast. In fact, I have often wondered if fasting could be used as a test to see if a person is eating incompatible foods. For those who fast and feel better, my guess would be that they are eating incorrectly, so not poisoning themselves three time a day is a definite improvement. This is yet another case of the diet gurus defining something (fasting) as healthy. But healthy as compared to what (eating the SAD diet)? In the case of the Original Diet, because it is naturally toxin free, fasting is counterproductive and certainly not what MA had in mind. For PA, food deprivation for any but a short length of time would be fatal, and it seems to me that fasting would put the body into a major state of stress.

Chapter 6 - Deviating From the Tier One Diet

In this section, we will look at communities around the world that deviate in one way or another from the Tier One Original Diet and yet live a very healthy life. The objective is to derive some clues to this phenomenon that may be applicable to our own lives, as well as assessing the potential health risks involved.

We all know people who seem to be able to eat "anything" and remain healthy, and they were referred to as the *winners* in the introduction section of this book. How are they able to do this? We can glimpse the answer by reviewing the findings of Weston Price as he went around the globe in the 1930s visiting indigenous tribes in an effort to determine how they stayed healthy. His conclusion was they ate local foods, the ones Nature had provided, which had been consumed in that same area by their ancestors for generations. Note, however, that these so-called primitive tribes were nowhere near as primitive as our PA. They all had the use of fire for cooking, and most had learned to fish, cultivate crops, and/or domesticate animals. By our definition, they certainly were not Ancient, and ate non-Original Diet foods while remaining healthy.

The diets of each of the healthy groups Price studied were all quite different. In the Swiss village where Price began his investigations, the inhabitants lived on whole rye bread and cheese, eaten with fresh milk of goats or cows. Meat was eaten about once a week, along with bone broth soups and a few vegetables they could cultivate during the short summer months. They were all healthy and had near perfect dentition, which was one of Price's yardsticks for determining health. Hearty Gallic fishermen (and presumably women) living off the coast of Scotland consumed no dairy products, and fish formed the mainstay of their diet, along with oats made into porridge and oatcakes. The Eskimo diet was composed largely of fish, roe, and marine animals, including seal oil and blubber.

Hunter-gatherers in Canada, the Everglades, the Amazon, Australia and Africa consumed game animals, particularly the parts that we tend to avoid, such as organ meats, blood, and marrow along with a variety of grains, tubers, vegetables and fruits that were available. African cattle-keeping tribes like the Masai consumed no plant foods at all--just meat, blood, and milk. South-sea islanders and the Maori of New Zealand ate lots of seafood along with pork meat and fat, and a variety of plant foods including coconut, cooked cassava root, and fruit. Insects were another common food in all regions except the Arctic. In sum, the range of foods that enabled the people he visited to remain healthy covered the gamut including meat with its fat, organ meats, whole milk products, fish, insects, whole grains, tubers, vegetables and fruit. How can this be reconciled with the relatively spartan Original Diet?

Enter Darwin. Let's start with the Swiss village Price first visited, which had about 2000 inhabitants at that time. The village was in a remote area of the Alps known as the Loetschental Valley, about a mile above sea level. We can safely imagine that these folks did not magically appear here, but migrated from lower, more populated areas of Switzerland. The fact that they had mastered grain cultivation, milling, and bread baking, along with animal domestication and milking practices would indicate quite a recent legacy, say within the last four thousand years. This is based on an estimate of the time of migration of grain eating from the Middle East (about 10,000 years ago) to its appearance in Western Europe some time in the Bronze Age. The valley had limited grazing area so it is unlikely it could have supported sufficient grazing animals to feed 2000 people on a meat diet, and the short growing season severely curtailed the availability of edible plants such as fresh fruit. Therefore, in order to survive, animal milking (as opposed to slaughter) would have been the intelligent approach, along with grain storage (to tide them over in the winter months).

Now, let us suppose that among the pioneering group that trekked into the valley generations ago was a group (or a family) that was intolerant of casein (a major milk protein) and/or gliadin (a major rye protein). How long do you think they would last on a milk/rye diet? This is where evolution takes over, and the survival of the fittest (those who, through evolution, can best fit into the environment) is the rule. The bottom line is that only those who, through evolution since the time of the Original Diet, acquired the ability to assimilate safely dairy and glutinous grains, and thus survived in this valley. All of the others died out.

Because of the isolation of the valley, there would have been considerable interbreeding, further enhancing the gene pool necessary to survive in this environment. What Price encountered was a group that had evolved to eat a dairy/grain diet, and hence thrived on it. It is very important to distinguish this conclusion from one that infers his discovery meant that a raw dairy/whole-grain diet is healthy for *all*. Many others and I can tell you from first hand experience that it most certainly is not and, if a person's heritage is not aligned with these foods, they can make one very ill indeed. In the case of the unlucky Swiss group, certain families became extinct. We can go down the list of every group that Price visited, and draw the same conclusions, with the only variable being the foods they ate, which were the ones necessary for survival in that particular environment.

Now, let's look at how this analysis translates into variations on the Original Diet. Clearly, since leaving Africa over a long period of emigration (guesses range from 50,000 to more than 1,000,000 years ago), PA was subjected to all sorts of environmental pressures that, over many generations of evolutionary variations, shaped the diet of his/her descendants to one that, out of necessity, may have been quite different from the Original Diet. This brings us to the present conundrum of finding the diet variations that each of us has acquired. If we knew that both sides of our family tree were direct descendants of the Loetschental Valley Swiss, we could decide with reasonable certainty that dairy and rye (and undoubtedly mountain spring water full of minerals) are healthy for us to eat and drink. Unfortunately, for most of us in the melting pot that represents a good part of modern Western civilization, it is rare that such a monolithic ancestry is the case.

Nutritionists have struggled with this question for a very long time, and from their efforts has emerged what can best be described as a hodge-podge of dietary advice based on such diverse personal characteristics as one's blood type, body type, metabolic type, genotype, Ayurvedic type, etc. I heard a skeptic in the field predict the development of a nutritional program based on one's social security number! As an avid experimenter, I enthusiastically and personally evaluated as many of these diets as I could find before deciding that I did not intend to place my future health in the hands of any of these programs. As Mark Twain so eloquently put it, be careful about reading health books– you may die of a misprint. The basis of most of these programs is that there is not one diet that fits all, but of course, I disagree. From my research, the Original Diet originally (and still does) fit all, and then some became acclimated to variations thereof, but none of us lost the ability to thrive on the original diet, which is quite a different conclusion.

Can we find any clues from MA on this subject? Well, from a look at the animal kingdom, it seems clear that virtually every other mammalian species on the planet has one natural diet that fits all, regardless of their location. Felines, from tigers to house cats, are natural obligate carnivores, whether in California or Africa, and they have three different blood types. Canines, from dogs to wolves, have at least 13 blood types, but all are natural carnivores. In the case of cattle, (where it seems that each distinct animal has its own blood type!), they are all naturally grass eating, whether in India or Indiana. I want to make the point that the above diets are those found in a *natural* environment.

Could we artificially breed a vegan dog? Sure, and it might even be healthier than one fed the typical canned cooked or dry dog Frankenfood. The same is true for humans. As omnivores, we can eat almost anything, and some of us do. At the risk of being redundant, I want to point out again that the Original Diet has been derived as the original one, *but not the only one*, for all humans, as designed by Nature. Individuals can modify or ignore it to their heart's content, with varying degrees of success, from perfect health to illness. I follow it for the simple reason that I do not like the odds of experimenting with other diets where my evolutionary compatibility with them is unknown, as is their impact on my health.

Ah, you may ask, isn't it possible that as a result of evolutionary adaptation to various diets, the Original Diet may no longer work for some of us? Can we lose our ability to assimilate animal foods and fruits? There are examples where nature has removed from us the ability to produce or properly assimilate certain foods or nutrients when it became evolutionarily unnecessary or inefficient to do so. One example is the ability to make Vitamin C, which we and other primates lack, presumably because we get enough from our diet. It is estimated that we lost this ability several million years ago, and it is not reversible. Lactose intolerance is caused by the loss of a digestive enzyme, lactase, as we reach adulthood, but there is some evidence that this intolerance may be reversible for some with prolonged ingestion of milk products. Although not related to food, our ability to make melanin in our skin decreased over many generations as we acclimated to sunlight-reduced environments far from the Equator, and this is not easily reversed.

The pattern here seems to be one of "use it or eventually lose it," with the unknown factor being the definition of "eventually." I do not know of any studies directed to answering the question of how long is long enough for permanent digestive changes, so let's see if we can get any clues from MA in this area. We will start by looking at the probability that humans can lose the ability to digest meat, say because they have lived a vegan lifestyle. Permanent genetic changes of the type we are talking about do not occur within a lifetime, but take many generations, so now we need to look at the possibility of multigenerational veganism.

From the research that Price conducted, virtually all of the native tribes he visited around the world were meat eaters, at least for a part of their diet. Some modern African tribes such as the Kikuyu and Wakamba were multi-generational agriculturists and their diet consisted of sweet potatoes, corn, beans, bananas, millet, or sorghum. However, there is also evidence that these tribes did consume large amounts of insects including flies, bees, wasps, beetles, butterflies, moths, crickets, dragonflies and termites, most of which are rich in the fat soluble factors found in blood, organ meats, fish and butterfat, which may have kept their digestive system attuned to animal protein and fats. Nevertheless, it is possible that if a person's heritage is from either of these tribes, or they know that both sides of their family have been healthy vegans for many generations, they theoretically may have lost the ability to digest properly animal fats and proteins, and perhaps should continue with a vegan lifestyle. Otherwise, it would seem that most of us have not been distanced from animal products for a sufficient period of time (multiple generations) that would permanently compromise our ability to digest them if we chose to do so.

I occasionally meet people that tell me they have a hard time digesting meat. It feels like it is sitting in their stomachs as a lump or is constipating, and makes them feel uncomfortable. Many of them assume that meat is just not a healthy food for them, which seems to be in conflict with the Original Diet. I will not be so arrogant as to state that everyone must eat meat to stay healthy, but I will present here a very analogous situation with our furry friends, our domesticated cats and dogs, as a possible lesson from Nature regarding the eating of meat.

My wife and I love cats, and as I write this book, we have two beautiful Tonkinese in-house cats that are tenth-generation raised eating raw animal food (meat, glands and other organs, and bones) and a very small amount of vegetable matter (from the guts of their prey) to match closely their native diet as carnivores. The breeder of these cats, Celeste Yarnall, has undertaken the task of raising cats on this diet in place of commercial pet food to demonstrate the health benefits for domesticated animals raised on a natural diet [73]. Considering the explosion of medical specialties in the veterinarian community (oncologists, dermatologists, radiologists, endocrinologists, etc.), and how it mirrors the human illness maintenance industry, her work is most timely. It also provides some interesting insights into issues we, who are also domesticated animals, may face in converting from a prepared food diet to a natural one.

Commercial cat food is filled with ingredients no undomesticated cat would normally ever eat, and it is then cooked, which destroys amino acids necessary for cat survival, such as taurine, which are added back in synthetic form. Remarkably, cats raised on this stuff no longer recognize or are attracted to their natural diet. Certainly, cats can survive for many years and reproduce on this Frankenfood, thanks to the miracles of science, but look at the illnesses they accumulate along the way, just like with humans.

Let us say you were given a cat that had been raised (perhaps for many generations) on commercial food and the task was to reintroduce her/him to their natural diet. (A vet once confided in me the obvious: the perfect food for a cat is a rat.) Well, it turns out this is no simple task. If you merely switch one food for another, the cat may stop eating and get quite ill. If you put the cat in the garden to catch a mouse, she/he may catch one and merely play with it, not knowing how to eat it. (This is traditionally learned from a hunting mother.) If you try force-feeding the cat, it may regurgitate the food or develop diarrhea. Some human companions might give up at this point, and conclude that the cat has lost its ability to eat its native diet. However, those dedicated to the task have found this is just not so. While it may be that certain digestive processes have gone into hibernation as unnecessary for the digestion of the commercial stuff, all is not lost. The trick that works is to start introducing the natural food in very small quantities along with the junk food, and slowly increase the amount, weaning the animal back to Nature, which could take some time, perhaps months. The effort is worth it – a cat on its way to leading a healthy natural life.

Sure, humans are not cats, but I presume the analogy to the above is now obvious; for those who want to experiment with meat but are concerned about the ability to digest it, one approach is to follow the cat program with a slow introduction. In a later section, I will also discuss some supplements that can be taken during the transition period to support the gut.

Finally, I would like to make a prediction for our modern society, based on Price's work. Using the theory postulated above that a society will, through selection, distill or cull its heritage to match its environment, including food, it would seem self-evident that the same culling is going on as you read this book. In other words, the health crises we are seeing today are in some part due to adaptation to the SAD diet. Those not evolved to handle it are in fact dying out, just like what happened in the Swiss village. That leaves those who, through the luck of heritage, are able to use these foods and will be the final victors in the health arena. This dying out process is taking the form of many of the chronic illnesses ravaging society, spurred on by our contaminated environment. Thanks to the miracles of medicine, we are able to stay alive, and hence able to reproduce more evolutionary losers (among whom I include myself), so this selection process is taking a very long time.

This presents an interesting race to see who will win – medical technology or MA. If history is any guide, MA always wins, leading to the result that future generations will be those adapted to eat cake, soda, candy, and French fries, and they will live long and healthy lives. In the meantime, in spite of the pressures from the food industry and the health community to fit into an environment for which I am not adapted, I am doing what I can to live a lifestyle that is in concert with the ancient heritage of my species, which of course, is the foundation of The Original Diet.

Chapter 7 - Foods Excluded From Tier One

The objective of this section is to look at the major food categories that were excluded from the Tier One Original Diet, in the context of the rationales for their exclusion. We will also try to estimate the degree of risk associated with adding a category into the diet. Table 3 is a list of the Tier Two and Three categories to be examined.

Anyone can add some or all of these foods to the Original diet to form for themselves a custom diet. I am presenting some of the criteria that a reader might want to consider in making such choices. As I have mentioned several times earlier in the book, each of us is responsible for our own food choices. Knowing the Original Diet and MA's plans can go a long way in making those choices informed ones.

Table 3

Tier Two and Tier Three Food Groups

Tier Two Foods

- Fish
- Fowl
- Eggs

Tier Three Foods

- Dairy
- Plant Parts Other Than Fruit (Seeds, Beans, Nuts, Tubers, Roots, Flowers, Leaves)
- Sugars (natural or artificial)
- Extracted Vegetable Oils
- Liquids Other Than Mineral/Spring Water

Chapter 8 - Tier Two Foods

The foods in this category were chosen because they would have passed the ABC test except that it is believed they were either not introduced until after cooking was available or not introduced until after the end of or very late in the Paleo era, primarily because of the physical difficulty in obtaining them. When they became available to PA, no significant processing was required, and they could be eaten raw.

Fish

The estimates for the introduction of fishing into our heritage range from about 125,000 to 20,000 years ago. It seems logical that shellfish would have been introduced into the diet first for those PA's near the sea, followed by the development of fishing. Note that both fish and shellfish are on the list of the most prevalent allergenic foods, which may be because of their late introduction into the diet.

Fish is a wonderful food nutritionally, and I would heartily suggest including it into an expanded Original Diet, except for the contamination issues. As most of you are aware, fish have become the leading source of environmental exposure to mercury. They absorb the toxic mineral from water as it passes over their gills and from eating other marine organisms. Large predator fish get an even higher dose from their prey – other fish. Mercury binds tightly to proteins in fish tissue, including muscle and, over time, it builds up in a process called bioaccumulation. Fish also accumulate toxic organic compounds such as PCBs (polychlorinated biphenyls), as do shellfish, which accumulate mercury at slightly lower levels than finfish. Compounding the organic toxin problem is that brominated flame-retardants known as PBDEs are everywhere and are quite toxic to humans. A study has shown that the neurotoxic effects of PBDEs are enhanced when combined with PCBs, such as found in fish [74].

Cooking fish does not reduce the toxin content, but does bring up another issue. One of the reported nutritional benefits of fish is the omega-3 fatty acid content. This fatty acid group is polyunsaturated and easily degraded by light, heat, and air (see the section below on essential fatty acids). Therefore, the ideal way to eat fish, for those who are going to eat it, is raw - sushi and sashimi are examples.

Eating fish is a Catch-22, and as discussed in *The Wellness Project*, the contaminants in fish are the very ones that many of us need to evict from our body to ensure health. The FDA has tried to define safe limits, but from my studies and hands-on experience in the world of detoxification, these limits are somewhat meaningless, arbitrary, and driven by industry. In the case of mercury alone, there is no test to measure total body burden in a human, and when you consider the added mercury burden from vaccinations and amalgam fillings, eating fish raises definite risks.

Now, let's look at the benefits of eating fish. The one most often referenced is the high content of omega-3 fatty acids, which are essential to the body. Comparing the omega-3 content of salmon with *grass-fed* beef yields a surprising result. Beef, on average, has slightly more omega-3 fatty acids by weight than fish (2% vs. 1.2%). It is also well known that the critical factor in essential fatty acids for humans is the ratio of omega-6 to omega-3 fatty acids. The ideal ratio is somewhere between 1:1 and 4:1, but for the SAD diet, the ratio can be over 20:1 due to an omega-6 overload. In the Original Diet, virtually the entire omega-6 overload has been eliminated, so that eating grass-fed meat easily achieves the desired fatty acid ratio without the need to consume any fish. Well, what about cholesterol – isn't the level in fish lower than that in meat? No, it is not, another surprise. The cholesterol level by weight for salmon is slightly higher than that for beef (as I previously indicated, the whole cholesterol issue is a *red herring* as far as I am concerned). Want more omega-3s? Eat organic grass-fed beef or lamb liver, which is loaded with good stuff [75].

Those who want to eat fish might want to concentrate on the smaller variety, because the smaller the fish the less contamination. As an example, sardines have a lower level of mercury than the large predators, but most commercially prepared sardines are canned, which is a less than healthy way of preparing fish. To meet health department requirements, canned fish must be essentially sterilized in the can to destroy all bacteria, which is why they last so long on the shelf. The time/temperature settings for this sterilization vary somewhat but are usually higher than the boiling point of water for many minutes. All of this takes place in a sealed metal can that may outgas its own toxins at these temperatures. As mentioned above, fragile omega-3 fats are easily damaged by heat, even though most of the air is evacuated from the can prior to heating. Thus, I cannot get too excited over a diet that includes canned fish (or canned anything, for that matter). Canning allows a product to sit on a shelf for years, which is good for the product's shelf life, but what about the shelf life of the consumer - does it contribute to their health and longevity? There are sources of salmon and other fish on the market that are selected for a lower than average mercury content, such as Vital Choice Wild Seafood [76].

This is a good place to mention other foods from the sea, such as algae in the form of seaweeds like kelp. Most of these are heavily contaminated with mercury, arsenic, and chemical toxins. The arsenic level in certain seaweed has gotten so high that there have been cases of arsenic poisoning in those eating large quantities [77]. Allergic reactions to fish can manifest as hives or swelling, or can be so serious that they are life-threatening. Fish proteins cause some of the symptoms, and worms or algae-based toxins cause others. As is the case for most allergic reactions to animal products, the symptoms appear very soon after eating the offending food. Fish oils and fish liver oils are discussed below in the section on essential fatty acids.

It is with a great deal of sadness that I take the position that until we can clean up the oceans, lakes, and rivers, I am staying away from anything presently living in these bodies of water. I take full responsibility for any personal bias in this decision, resulting from my own horrific mercury toxicity experience, due in part to my love of fish. I am not suggesting that all others follow suit. I feel quite confident that there are many people that can ingest loads of mercury and PCBs without health consequences.

Fowl

Somewhere along the timeline—we don't know quite when—humans learned how to catch and eat birds. Chickens are a domesticated bird descended from the red junglefowl, or guineafowl, related to the pheasant, of which there is an African variety. The flesh can be safely eaten raw, assuming the fowl is truly free range, and organically fed. The best guess as to domestication is about 1500 BCE by the Egyptians, which is extremely recent. The modern turkey is not related to chickens, and it appears to be native to North or Central America. Other flying birds native to Africa are duck and goose, and for the non-purist, these would be my first choices for experimental additions to the Original Diet because of their high fat content. As a caution, chicken is high on the list of allergens, perhaps due to its more recent introduction into our diet. Symptoms of bird allergy usually show up very soon after eating and may include rashes, stomachache, fatigue, headache, and respiratory problems. I personally love duck and eat it on occasion. For those who are fowl lovers, I strongly recommend selecting organically fed free-range birds, which are readily available in health food markets.

Eggs

Eggs might fit closer to the acceptable time-line category simply because hunter-gatherers could easily climb up trees to a certain height and raid nests, so eggs would have been available earlier than the birds themselves (who were much harder to catch). Ostrich eggs may have been the earliest obtained as food in this category, since ostrich nests are in the ground.

Nutritionally, eggs are a great food choice, especially if eaten raw, assuming they are from organically- fed free-range birds. Raw retains the full, undamaged value of the fatty acids and prevents oxidation of the cholesterol in the yolk. While salmonella is a concern, statistics show that such contamination is very rare. A strong defense system (which is a goal of The Original Diet) is intended to handle the bacteria with perhaps a stomachache or the runs as the toxins are eliminated. If raw is not appealing (it does not appeal to me), cook eggs as gently as possible, boiling or poaching them to protect the fatty acids. The temperatures involved in frying are much higher than boiling and likely to cause fatty acid damage in ways we have yet to determine.

Some people, including me, are allergic to egg albumen, which is part of the white of the egg. A simple saliva test can sometimes pick up antibodies to albumen, and taking one may be worth it for those who choose to add eggs to the Original Diet [78]. Allergic symptoms to eggs are very similar to those of chicken allergy. In my case, I toss the whites and only eat the yolks, without any symptoms. Actually, I would discourage eating egg whites without the yolks, particularly if the whites are raw. The whites contain avidin, a protein that bind up biotin, an important vitamin. On the other hand, egg yolks are very rich in biotin, and I do not know of any adverse effects of eating only the yolks. Personally, I love medium-boiled egg yolks and eat them often. I choose high omega-3 eggs from organically fed free-range birds fed high omega-3 natural foods such as flax seeds. There is more detail on this topic in the essential fatty acid section below.

Now, onward to a discussion of the Tier Three foods.

Chapter 9 - Tier Three Foods

The Tier Three foods are the ones that were excluded from the Original Diet because of potentially high levels of natural toxins. Aside from dairy, all of the other foods in this group are in the plant kingdom. There is no question in my mind that there are large numbers of people that can safely ingest many of these foods without compromising their health. The problem, of course, is the lack of knowledge as to which person fits which food. While I am very comfortable suggesting Tier One Foods, and also quite comfortable suggesting Tier Two foods (other than fish), because my research supports these food categories, I will not be so arrogant as to presume to have the answers when it comes to the Tier Three food category. At the end of this section, I will propose an approach that may lessen the impact of these foods on the defense system of those who wish to continue eating large amounts of Tier Three foods.

I have already suggested some pointers that might be of use in food selection, such as knowledge of one's dietary heritage over several generations of healthy ancestors on both sides of the family. Other pointers that may be of use come from our chimpanzee cousins. We know that at times when fruit was not readily available, those chimps with the intelligence to break open the shells of nuts did so and ate them as a source of nutrition, so freshly shelled raw nuts might be a category to investigate. On the other hand, roots and tubers seem to have exceedingly high levels of natural toxins, and chimpanzees are not known to eat much from this plant category.

Of course, cooking methods can have a great effect on natural toxins (increasing or decreasing them), so this is another variable to consider. For detailed discussions of various cooking methods and how they may relate to toxins, I want to again recommend the book *Nourishing Traditions* by Sally Fallon, as well as the food-related articles that appear on the Weston A. Price website [17] [7].

Another factor that can have a major impact on Tier Three food choices is the present nutritional status of the individual. As an example, it is one thing to eat plant foods that tend to bind minerals and prevent their absorption when you already have high minerals levels. The health impact of occasionally eating these foods would likely be minimal. On the other hand, if your present nutritional status is such that you are already mineral deficient, eating these same foods could have a substantial impact on health. As you will see from a reading of the detox chapter, unnatural toxins in the body have a strong impact on nutritional status, which is why I do not believe one can separate diet from detoxification in any meaningful way on the road to health. Therefore, I think it is prudent for the reader to become familiar with the toxin issues discussed in *The Wellness Project* before deciding on dietary choices.

Most tests for food incompatibilities look for some immune system response to ingesting the proteins or other compounds in these foods. The result of such testing is often a false negative (indicating you are not intolerant, when you really are), based on a number of variables. One is when you last ate that food. Another is the total length of time you have been eating that food, and finally there is the condition of your immune system to consider. If you have not eaten the suspected food lately, there may be no measurable immune system response. If you have been eating that food for a very long time, the immune system may no longer respond to its toxic compounds, and this also can be the case if your immune system is in a weakened state. I know of people who tested negative for a variety of foods, yet when they eliminated them from their diet as a trial, their health improved. This indicates to me that an elimination diet, where potentially incompatible foods are not eaten for, say, a few months, may be the best way to make some food choices. Armed with the information in this section, it would be easy to use the Tier One diet as the baseline, eliminating Tier Two and Tier Three foods in a planned manner and noting the result. This approach can work well for those foods where the negative response (or its absence) is easy to detect and occurs in a reasonable time period. Other than the above, I do not know of any foolproof way to evaluate food choices, which is why I take the easy way out and stick mostly to the Tier One foods.

As I now go through each of the categories of foods in Tier Three, I will attempt to suggest approaches that may be of assistance in the food consumption decision-making process.

Dairy

Humans are the only mammals that routinely drink the milk of another mammal, and do so into adulthood. I don't presume to know Nature's plans, but this sure does not sound like one of them. The introduction of milking would have taken place some time after cattle domestication, believed to have begun about 10-12,000 years ago in the Middle East. The economic advantages are obvious. You can get a lot more protein and fat from a cow by milking it for as long as possible as opposed to killing it for food, and this undoubtedly was the original motivation for consuming dairy. It is interesting that some indigenous African tribes visited by Weston Price had developed an alternate approach to this problem by drinking small amounts of cow blood over time, while keeping the cow alive.

Assuming we are not under the environmental pressure of having to drink milk or starve, let us look at the pros and cons of dairy as an addition to the Original Diet. Referring now to unpasteurized and non-homogenized milk as it comes from a free-range organically grown grass-fed cow that has been spared hormones and antibiotics, the pros are that it is a good source of animal protein and fat, as well as fat-soluble vitamins. While milk is supposedly a good source of calcium, most of it is not very available to the bones because of missing co-factors, including magnesium, and this calcium can build up in the arteries unless there is enough magnesium present. I regard magnesium deficiency as a major factor in the near-epidemic osteoporosis scare among women, and it is covered in detail in the magnesium factor section below. Milk can be fermented and otherwise processed into a variety of foods such as cheese, yogurt, and kefir, some of which are high in supposedly healthy bacteria, and it can be churned into butter. For those readers who are fortunate enough to have a heritage that is compatible with dairy, as long as sufficient magnesium is in the diet, dairy is a reasonably good food source. For the rest of us, it is not.

Well, how does a person know if they are dairy compatible? Going back to the groups visited by Price as an example, he found several that thrived on dairy, including our Swiss friends, who needed it to support their population. Once again, for those who know their heritage on both sides for many generations, and it fits one of these indigenous populations, I would say their chances of dairy compatibility are high. There is also some evidence that portions of Northern European countries have subsisted for generations on dairy (for the same reasons of survival), and this may be a clue that you can include dairy in your diet if that is your heritage. Tests have shown that the majority of the adult populations in these areas are still able to produce lactase, an enzyme necessary to break down the milk sugar lactose.

However, estimates are that 70-80% of the world's adult population is lactose intolerant, having lost the lactase enzyme on the way to adulthood (it is needed in children to digest breast milk). Well, I can take a hint from MA, and to me this is a big one. There are a variety of tests that can be performed to see if a person is lactose intolerant, and for some people it is obvious from the bloated feeling in their gut when they consume dairy. If no immediate adverse effects occur, does that mean compatibility? No. If tests show lactose tolerance, does that mean dairy tolerance? No. In addition to the sugar lactose, there are at least two animal proteins in milk that have been identified as troublesome to many humans, casein and whey, and there are some tests for intolerance to these as well.

Are there additional troublesome compounds in milk? Researchers are still trying to figure out what is in milk (human and otherwise), which is no easy task because it is filled with a multitude of compounds. Ignorance in this area has produced some embarrassing (and sometimes fatal) results in the infant formula business, where manufacturers periodically realize they have left something out that is critical to the health of a baby. What is known is that cow's milk is different from human milk, and is undoubtedly the perfect food for a calf. Some of the relatively immediate symptoms that an intolerant or allergic person might experience from dairy include nausea, diarrhea, bloating, flatulence, itchy skin, gastrointestinal upsets, excess mucus, and respiratory disturbances.

Of course, those that have a problem with dairy can try to fool Mother Nature by getting lactose-free milk or by taking enzymes, and some of the obvious symptoms may abate. From my perspective, fooling with MA is a risky business. I know people who stopped dairy and their respiratory problems and arthritic pain disappeared very quickly. There isn't a clear explanation, but dairy seems to stir up inflammatory responses in the body that disappear when the dairy disappears.

For those who want to experiment with dairy, I strongly suggest getting products that most closely resemble what Nature intended, not an easy task. A starting point is to avoid pasteurization, homogenization, reduced-fat products, growth-hormones, antibiotics, grain-fed animals, and vitamin D2 supplementation, all of which turn milk into Frankenmilk. This leaves a precious few family-run dairies that avoid all of these pitfalls and sell raw milk and milk products. Unfortunately, they periodically run afoul of regulatory agencies that want to put them out of business, ostensibly for selling an unhealthy product! Their concern is that the milk will be contaminated with bacteria because it is not pasteurized, and I address this issue below. A grass-roots effort has been underway to lobby regulatory agencies to try to keep alive the right to access raw milk [79]. For those who are tolerant of dairy, this is an important project to support. In any case, I suggest that dairy eaters supplement with magnesium to avoid an overload of unusable and potentially harmful calcium. Note that the synthetic vitamin D2 supplementation added to some dairy products interferes with magnesium absorption (vitamin D3 is the correct form to use).

This is probably a good place to discuss pasteurization. What we know from a nutritional standpoint is that pasteurizing milk (or any other food) is not a good idea. The bulk of commercial dairy available in the world is pasteurized, a process that unfortunately creates toxicity. Dairy food requires the very bacteria that pasteurization kills to make it digestible for those who can digest it, and to suppress other bacteria toxic to humans. Pasteurization actually renders milk more toxic with time because it no longer contains the beneficial bacteria needed to control overgrowth of toxins. At least one of these bacteria is of the spore-forming type discussed earlier.

The reasons we have pasteurization have to do with money. The first reason is that the supply chain from cow to consumer is filthy, and it costs money to clean it up. By filthy, I mean it is contaminated with bacteria and other pathogens that can make one sick. The problem begins with the cows themselves. In most dairies, they are kept in unnaturally close quarters, and given antibiotics in their feed along with growth hormones. The result is a chemical cow with disturbed gut flora. The cow problem is so bad that cow dung is now toxic, and when it is used intentionally or unintentionally to fertilize vegetables (like spinach), they too become toxic with pathogens such as E.coli. This may surprise some readers, but cow dung from healthy cows (free-range, grass-fed, no hormones or antibiotics) has antibiotic properties and is an insect repellant! In India, it is used topically as part of Ayurvedic medicine to treat skin problems. It is also used as a floor liner to repel insects, particularly mosquitoes, and of course, it is a great fertilizer [80].

The second reason for pasteurization also has to do with money. By destroying much of the beneficial bacteria and enzymes, pasteurization extends the shelf life of products dramatically, resulting in significant cost savings compared to raw products. Virtually all liquid foods in a can or bottle and many in sealed boxes are pasteurized, which causes a loss of vitamins and enzymes, resulting in Frankendrinks.

The pasteurization process was popularized by Pasteur, as was the germ theory and vaccinations, although according to several historians, he did not develop any of these himself. During his lifetime, the Germ Theory (germs cause disease, leading to the conclusion that they need to be killed to stop disease) was in competition with what is called the Terrain Theory, which taught that defects in the internal environment of the body permit germs to cause illness, and that strengthening this internal environment is the key to health. I discuss this competition of theories and its consequences in much more detail in The Wellness Project.

Returning to the dairy discussion, some people that have an adverse reaction to Frankenmilk feel better with raw milk products from properly treated range-fed cows, and others feel better using fermented dairy products such as yogurt or kefir. In fact, there are isolated communities that thrive on these products, such as those in mountainous areas of Eastern Europe, including Bulgaria and the Caucauses, and they live very long and healthy lives. Once again, if a person's heritage is well known, they might feel confident enough to add these products to their diet. I personally do not feel good eating any raw dairy, fermented or not, which is too bad because I really love cheese. Although it would be helpful if I could enumerate all of the adverse long and short-term effects of eating dairy if it is not in a person's evolutionary makeup to do so, there is insufficient information for a comprehensive list. One problem is the long time lapse between ingestion and symptoms, leading to a cause-effect disconnect.

Some relevant information may be gleaned from a study performed in China where rural Chinese people who consumed dairy foods high in the protein casein developed major illnesses over time. The Chinese people have a long history of not eating dairy, so the outcome of this study is no surprise, and clearly shows the long-term effects of a dietary evolution/environment mismatch. The author of the study came to the conclusion that the solution to the problem is to adopt a vegan diet, discounting the possibility that eating the proper animal foods (i.e. the Original Diet) might produce the best overall health result [81].

On a personal note, I went through an experimental phase a few years ago where I introduced a lot of raw cheese into my diet. After several weeks, I developed heel pain that was quite annoying, and which I never had experienced before. Upon stopping the cheese, it resolved in about a week. Months later, I repeated the experiment (I am sometimes a glutton for punishment) with the same result. I thought at the time that the high calcium content of the cheese was somehow causing my problem by displacing magnesium. More recently, while running some experiments with various mineral combinations, I was able to reproduce the heel pain whenever I took high doses of calcium without offsetting it with similarly high doses of magnesium. I now feel comfortable stating that excessive intake of calcium, as may happen with a high dietary intake of dairy, can be a cause of bone spurs if it is accompanied by a magnesium deficiency. As discussed at length in the mineral section below, magnesium deficiency may arise in those people leading a chronically stressful life, because stress rapidly depletes magnesium. This leads me to the conclusion that those modern societies that do well on a high dairy intake in their diet also must have a reliable source of dietary magnesium, and a lifestyle that is low in chronic stress. One source of magnesium could be mineral water, or maybe people in these societies have developed the ability to extract magnesium from plant parts such as nuts and seeds, somehow overcoming the natural toxins such as phytates and oxalates that interfere with mineral assimilation for many of us.

That brings me to a discussion of calcium, considered by the dairy industry as one of the important ingredients in milk products, particularly for bone health. Further, we are all told by mainstream and alternative health communities and the government RDA (Recommended Daily Allowance) charts that we need at least 1000 mg of calcium daily. Since the Original Diet (and that of our ancestors for 99,600 generations) does not include dairy, let's check in with MA to see if she can shed any light on the subject. From ancient skeletons and teeth, we know that PA had excellent bone strength, on average better that modern man. From a survival point of view, this would make sense since a hunter-gatherer with a broken bone was probably a goner. Of course, these skeletons were all from a period where animals had not yet been domesticated (a recent event), and hence dairy was not part of our ancestral diet for about 2.45

million years. So, where did PA get his supposedly "necessary" 1000 mg of calcium?

Before we try to answer this question, let's take a look at the RDAs for nutrients, since many diet plans use the RDA as a standard. The RDA is put together by a governmental committee, and is supposed to be based on averages derived from "healthy people." It is not updated very often. *Healthy* is certainly a relative term, but you can be assured it is based on people who eat the SAD diet, including all of the categories of foods not included in the Original Diet. The Tier Three plant foods in particular contain anti-nutrients such as phytates (in grains, nuts and seeds) that are known to interfere with the assimilation of minerals, including calcium and magnesium. Oxalate is another plant anti-nutrient found in such vegetables as spinach and rhubarb and in most grains, and it also binds calcium and magnesium [82]. Therefore, one can conclude that a person eating foods high in these and other anti-nutrients would end up requiring a much higher mineral intake than one on an anti-nutrient-free diet like the Original Diet.

If that were the case, the RDA of 1000 mg might be reduced to, say, 600 mg for those on the Original Diet. I give this example to illustrate that the RDA system presently in place is likely to be largely irrelevant for our purposes, and in fact, I do not know of any studies to determine what the "real" numbers are. To compound the problem, it is also very difficult even to determine the micronutrient nutritional value of the Original Diet as it would have appeared to PA. This is because the nutritional values we presently use, generated by the USDA, reflect present-day food products, which in many instances are vastly different (lower) than the nutritional content of those foods in the time of PA because of soil depletion and other modern agricultural issues.

From my review of the literature, most of the plant nutrient falloff between PA's time and today has occurred in the vegetable category as opposed to fruit, but there is no good database that I am aware of that tracks this information. Of course, much of it is lost because we have no record of the composition of most ancient plant products. The point is, we may have to add food supplements in certain categories, somewhat based on guesswork, with the goal in mind of restoring the Original Diet to its original nutritional value. As you will see in a later discussion, it is my opinion that PA obtained a major portion of his/her dietary calcium (and magnesium) intake from natural mineral water, which you will recall is an important element of the Original Diet. Animal blood is another source. There are about 5 grams of calcium in the blood alone of a typical cow [18], along with about 750 mg of magnesium [83].

A discussion of calcium usually brings up the topic of osteoporosis (porous bone), which today is the major driving force behind high-dose calcium. Let's start with defining the goal in the "war against osteoporosis," which is the prevention of bone fragility that can lead to frequent fractures. In other words, we want *strong* bones. What does bone strength have to do with osteoporosis? In many instances, nothing. I remember taking a course in school called Strength of Materials, where we learned early on that there in not necessarily a direct correlation between material strength and its density, or its porosity, or its hardness. A key factor for strength is the crystal structure of the material.

Bone mineral density is typically measured using dual-energy x-ray absorptiometry, known as the DEXA test. It is supposed to yield a measure of osteoporosis, a term that seems to have many definitions, but the objective of the test is to determine risk of fracture. In fact, however, one can test as having osteoporosis, yet have very strong bones that are not at all likely to fracture. On the other hand, one can test as having excellent bone density, yet have fragile bones very prone to fracture. So, what good is the test? Well, it sells a lot of drugs called bisphosphonates, which do increase bone density, so you pass the DEXA test, but unfortunately they can make your bones more fragile, whereby you are very prone to fracture [84]. In some very sad cases, the drugs actually cause bone disintegration, particularly of the jaw, which is somewhat impossible to repair [85].

On the other side of the coin, Inuits, who subsist on a diet of animal food that seems very low in calcium, test as having a high rate of osteoporosis, yet they have very low fracture rates, which puzzles the researchers [86]. In other words, they have a diet low in calcium, would fail the DEXA test, but have very strong bones. As you can imagine, for their lifestyle, frequent bone fractures would be catastrophic. As we will see later, this supposed puzzlement also occurs among menopausal Mayan women.

What can we make of this dilemma? The only way to definitively measure bone strength that I know of is destructive – testing how much force it takes to break the bone - so let's leave that out. What remains is a wait-and-see type of destructive test based on accidents – in other words, wait until you fall and see what happens. I do not like those odds, so I am betting that the Original Diet, tested by 99,000 generations will work for me. So far, so good. I have had some nasty spills over the last 20 years, but have never broken anything - yet. Note that some of the factors that have a positive influence on healthy bone are magnesium, vitamin D, and vitamin K. These nutrients are further discussed in the food supplement section. The effectiveness of calcium used alone as a supplement to strengthen bones has been discredited [87].

A discussion of dairy would not be complete without a discussion of infant formula. In theory, human milk is the ideal food for human babies and, of course, is in keeping with MA's design. I say in theory because it all depends on the health of the mother. In some instances, because of a lousy diet, the mother is deficient in important nutrients that are then also lacking in her milk. Another scenario is that the mother's body is loaded with toxins that pass through to her milk, toxifying the baby. One of the most insidious of these is mercury from amalgam fillings, vaccinations, fish, or all of the above (discussed in the detox section of *The Wellness Project*). For these and other reasons, it is sometimes necessary to find an alternative to mother's milk, which is no easy task, especially since we have yet to define all of its components. What is clear is that the composition of the milk of a different species (cow, goat, etc.) is different in many respects, and we really do not know what the long-term effects are on the health of a person raised on these products. Under any conditions, the substitute milk used should be raw, from grass-fed animals that are hormone and antibiotic free. Valiant efforts have been made by the alternative health community to try to design a human milk substitute, and examples can be found on the Weston Price Foundation website previously referenced [7].

Let's see if we can get any clues from MA. First, of course, it is important that a woman intending to get pregnant should first clean up her body with the right diet and detoxification protocols (see *The Wellness Project* for detox protocols). If problems remain in breastfeeding, the natural solution, which has been around for ages, is to substitute the human milk of another nursing mother either who has excess milk or who has weaned her baby but decided to act as a "wet nurse" to aid other mothers. There are many examples of this in the animal kingdom, where a nearby adult female sustains abandoned cubs, or even cubs of another species. There are several caveats to implementing this solution for humans. The first is that the surrogate must also be in good health with respect to diet and toxins. The second is how to get fresh human milk from one distant location to another without contamination or other damage. The last thing you want to do is to pasteurize the milk, which would kill a lot of the good stuff. Freezing may be a possibility. Well, these are not easy problems to solve, and very few people are working on them for the classic reason that there is really no money in it as compared to selling canned infant formula in the supermarket. Besides, it is inconvenient, so the Western world continues to fool with Mother Nature, with unknown consequences.

I want to bring up another and in my view more elegant, solution to this problem that is also ancient, which I will call the "grandmother solution." It is well known that non-pregnant women (even those in or post-menopause) can induce lactation through repeated nipple stimulation, either by placing a suckling child to the breast repeatedly or by using mechanical means. I consider this a very important clue from MA. Assuming one or more healthy grandmothers are locally available, this to me is a wonderful and natural solution to breast feeding problems, which would, incidentally, form strong baby-grandmother ties. For the adventurous grandmas out there, here is an interesting experiment right out of a rocket scientist's bag of tricks. There are a variety of electrically powered breast pumps on the market for nursing mothers [88]. The experiment I have in mind would be to hook one of those up to a willing participant as a nipple stimulator, using it on a daily basis to see if it can indeed induce lactation. By the way, fellows, MA has also provided men with the ability to lactate in response to nipple stimulation, so keep that in mind when your nursing wife is tired!

If you think about it, this is really a gift from MA to assist in the continuation of our species. One can imagine in the time of PA that many nursing mothers died for the typical reasons of starvation, predators, or accidents, and the ability of others in the family to continue breastfeeding the child would be in concert with the survival of the species. Modernly, it allows mothers of adopted children also to experience the wonders of breastfeeding. The La Leche League website has some discussions on inducing lactation [89].

This naturally brings me to the topic of menopause. Yes, menopause. If menopause is truly a natural phenomenon as opposed to one that is environmental in origin, its purpose remains one of MA's great mysteries. While I doubt that menopause should be characterized as an illness, its origins are quite unusual and it occurs rarely in other mammals. The two simplified explanations are that menopause is meant to protect the older female from the rigors of childbirth, and that animals don't live long enough to experience menopause. Maybe, but these are just guesses.

Here is what we presume to know from research, filtered by my personal interpretation. Each woman is born with a set number of eggs, apparently predetermined before birth, and it is believed that this pool of eggs is never replenished, which may or may not be the case. At around 16-20 weeks of gestation, a female fetus will have the greatest number of eggs (about 6-7 million). For unknown reasons, at birth, this number decreases to about 2 million, and by puberty to about 300,000. This process of decline continues throughout life until menopause, and does not seem to be interrupted by birth control pills, pregnancy, or ovulation. From this reservoir of eggs, fewer than 500 will ovulate during a woman's reproductive years, until they run out at menopause.

What does menopause have to do with dairy? Well, in the search for a reason for menopause, one colorful theory that has emerged is called the "grandmother hypothesis," and it goes something like this [90]. It is conceivable that during our evolutionary history, older mothers who lost their fertility were able to spend more of their time helping, protecting, and teaching their children and grandchildren. Experiments and observation have shown that those animals that have had time invested in them by family members, in the form of protection and education, are much more likely to live to the age at which they are able to reproduce, certainly a Natural goal. The reason I am bringing this up here is that the ability to induce lactation, even in a menopausal woman, may favor this theory just on the basis that it allows grandmothers to nurture, even years after the loss of fertility.

While on the subject of menopause, an interesting question to ponder is whether aligning one's heritage with one's lifestyle (particularly diet) would obviate the annoying symptoms of menopause without the need for hormone therapy. I can find two studies relating to the issue, both concerning Mayan women. The first study of a small group of Mayan women in the Yucatan found that none could recall any of the typical symptoms of menopause so prevalent in our society, such as hot flashes. Even though tests showed they had the typical menopausal decreases in bone density and estrogen, there was no increase in fractures or decrease in height [91]. A later study of Mayan women in the highlands of Guatemala found a higher incidence of reporting menopausal symptoms. The clearly puzzled author concluded that "symptoms in women in the years around menopause must be interpreted in geographical, nutritional, biological, psychological and cultural context" [92]. Other ethnic studies have also found puzzling differences between cultures. For example, there is no word for hot flashes in the Japanese language [93].

While I would like to think the Original Diet could have a major impact on menopause symptoms, I have only one case study – my wife. She is in menopause, uses no hormone therapy, and when she sticks somewhat closely to the Original Diet, she is symptom free. If she starts to deviate too much, hot flashes appear. She can control them to some extent by taking clay, which would indicate there is a toxin connection to some menopausal symptoms. Since it seems clear that PA favored animal glands and other organs, I wonder if the ovaries from prey animals were reserved for the women in the family. For adventuresome female readers with menopausal symptoms, an additional food supplement to the Original Diet might be an ovary glandular, such as Cytozyme-O by Biotics Research [94]. The bottom line for me regarding dairy is to avoid or minimize its consumption on the basis that the benefits of eating other-species dairy (if there are any) do not outweigh the risks.

For those who want to experiment with dairy and yet are unsure of their level of intolerance, gelatin, found in bone broth, has been found to improve the digestion of milk and milk products, particularly casein. Gelatin is discussed in detail in the food supplement section below.

Plant Parts Other Than Fruit

In this section, we are going to discuss seeds (grains), beans, nuts, tubers, roots, stems, flowers, and leaves. In many instances, I will be referring to human attempts to eliminate natural plant toxins by the use of heat, soaking, fermenting, etc., and the lack of efficacy of such attempts. While there are dozens of supporting references on the subject, a particularly useful one in this area is *Toxic Constituents of Plant Foodstuffs*, edited by Irvin Liener [31].

Grains

In the Original Diet discussion, we covered the basics of why portions of plants other than sweet fruit are not included. Here, we will look at a risk/benefit analysis for a variety of excluded plant products to evaluate the prudence of adding any of them to the Original Diet.

The glutinous grains (seeds) such as wheat, barley and rye have the most notoriety with respect to allergies and intolerances that may lead to delayed illnesses, ranging from aching joints, gastrointestinal disorders, depression, eczema, low blood iron levels, and an increased risk of diabetes, bowel cancer, anemia, and osteoporosis. Celiac disease is a gluten-related intestinal illness that interferes with the absorption of nutrients from food. This condition damages or destroys the tiny, fingerlike protrusions lining the intestines through which nutrients are absorbed into the bloodstream. While there are some gliadin antibody tests that might uncover this problem, I know of many cases of what seem to be false negatives, based on the fact that stopping the intake of grains for these people yielded great health improvements regardless of negative test results for grain intolerance.

From Price's research, we know that several modern indigenous groups in Western Europe have incorporated grains into their diet, such as the Swiss group (rye) and the Scottish group (oats). Starting about 10,000 years ago, the spread of grain consumption form the Middle East to Western Europe is estimated to have taken several thousand years. Therefore, in areas such as Switzerland and Scotland, grains are an even more recent crop, being incorporated into the diet say about 4000 years or about 160 generations ago. What this indicates to me is how quickly environmental pressure can cause evolutionary "selection" in monolithic communities, whereby those who by heritage are not able to accommodate the available foods die off, and the remainder thrives. As I indicated above, if a person can trace their heritage to these specific groups, their chances of compatibility to these respective grains may be quite good. However, as a caution, the modern populations of far Western Europe, particularly the British Isles, such as the Irish, British and Scottish, have an extremely high incidence of gluten intolerance, most likely because of the short period of adaptation [95]. Note that oats do not naturally contain gluten, but may become contaminated with it during harvesting and processing.

About 80% of the world's human population subsists on grains for want of other food sources, and their individual genetic heritage will undoubtedly determine their health outcome. Some of the non-glutinous grains in wide use are corn and rice, and there has been resurgence in the use of some ancient gluten-free grains, or pseudo-grains, such as the seeds and leaves of quinoa and amaranth. Quinoa contains saponins and is toxic raw (birds will not eat it). Amaranth, also toxic raw, is high in oxalates and the leaves are high in nitrates that can convert to toxic nitrites during heating. This is just more of the same story that Nature does not seem to want us tampering with her seeds. For those of us fortunate enough not to need to eat seeds for sustenance, there is no nutritional benefit to adding them to the Original Diet.

I love wheat, and as a kid, I could eat a loaf of rye bread and wash it down with a box of pretzels. What I did not know at that time was that wheat feeds Candida (discussed in detail in *The Wellness Project*), and I already had a severe overgrowth of this fungus as a result of frequent antibiotic use as a child. The bottom line for me: other than some brown rice occasionally, I don't go near any of this stuff. We have not even scratched the surface in identifying the toxins in these portions of plants, and I for one do not want to be a guinea pig in this arena when there is no health benefit.

For those who wish to have grains as part of their diet, I suggest avoiding the glutinous variety, as in wheat, rye, and barley, and concentrating instead on whole grain versions of brown rice, quinoa, and amaranth. You can experiment with fermentation and sprouting to try to lower the natural toxin content. Because virtually all corn is GMO, I avoid it. Presoaking oats can reduce its toxin levels somewhat. Sally Fallon's book *Nourishing Traditions* has lots of information in this area [17]. Another approach is the use of gelatin, found in bone broth, which has been found to improve the digestibility of the proteins in grains other than corn [96]. Gelatin is discussed in detail in the food supplement section below.

Beans

Beans are like seeds and Nature has taken great pains to protect them because they represent the reproductive potential for plants. Detoxifying efforts have been made, such as sprouting them, fermenting them, soaking them, and heating them, but none have been completely successful.

Most of us have participated in the jokes regarding eating beans and large volumes of intestinal gas, caused by complex sugar molecules called oligosaccharides that are broken down by the large intestine into carbon dioxide and hydrogen. The end result (pun intended) is gas, which I view as yet another graphic clue from MA that most of us are not adapted to digesting them as a result of a missing enzyme, very much like lactose intolerance for dairy. Sure, you can resort to Beano® and try to fool Mother Nature, but I don't know if you really are, and neither does anybody else.

A classic example of bean toxicity is soy, supposedly a health food, at least in the minds of the soy industry. I invite soy lovers to read the book *The Whole Soy Story*, by Kaayla Daniel [97]. I have yet to find a soy eater who has read this book and continued to eat any soy products. A wealth of information can also be found on the Weston Price Foundation website [7]. They have posted online a brochure called *Soy Alert!* that should do the trick. Reading the above literature will also give one great insight into the supposed love affair between the Asian culture and soy (historically, on average they eat about two teaspoons per day of naturally fermented soy as a condiment).

Because there is so much great information out there on the dangers of soy, I will not spend a lot of time on it here, except to hit a few highlights. The phytoestrogens in soy can disrupt the endocrine system, leading to testicular problems for young boys and early puberty in young girls, so using it in infant formula is really bad news (it travels in breast milk), and it can also contribute to breast cancer and infertility. High levels of phytic acid interfere with mineral assimilation, including calcium, possibly contributing to bone fractures. Trypsin inhibitors interfere with protein digestion and may cause pancreatic disorders. Goitrogens can cause hypothyroidism, autoimmune thyroid disease, and possibly thyroid cancer. The processing of soy to make the Frankenfoods you see in the market contributes to the production of highly carcinogenic nitrosamines.

For me, soy is a poster child as to why you do not want to fool with MA, at least in the bean category, which also includes peanuts. Peanuts are not a nut and are variously referred to as a bean, or a legume, or a pod, or a pulse, depending on a nightmare of definitions in this field, and are one of the most allergenic of foods.

Flax seed has become popular as a plant source of omega-3 fatty acids. Like most seeds, it must be processed to yield any nutritional value, since the whole seed would go right through your digestive system (as MA intended). Because of the fragile oil profile, once milled, it must be consumed quickly, and to avoid rancidity, never heated. Flaxseed contains some interesting anti-nutrients including very high levels of phytate, the mineral binder, and ones that interfere with vitamins B6 and B1.

For those who want to include beans in their diet, I would avoid soy unless it is traditionally fermented in the Japanese style, and then only eat it in small quantities. I would also favor those beans that can be eaten raw with minimal discomfort, such as snap and green beans. As in the case of grains, gelatin has been shown to increase the digestibility of the proteins in beans [96].

Nuts

One of the most popular nuts in Africa is the mongongo nut, which is a favorite of elephants because of its sweet fruit covering. The elephants are drawn to the sweet fruit, the nuts survive their digestive tract, and end up in heaps around the forest floor along with a pile of fertilizer, just as MA intended. Modern foragers harvest them from the heaps and heat them to open the very hard shells and get at the nut. If one can trace their heritage to Kalahari Bushmen, perhaps cooked mongongo nuts are right for them. Other than that, nuts suffer the same fate as seeds, where a variety of processing methods have been tried to reduce toxicity, with limited success. Some, such as the apricot kernel and bitter almond, are sufficiently toxic that their compounds are used as a drug (laetrile) in an attempt to kill cancer cells (some even suggest they cause cancer). They contain amygdalins, which produce cyanide. While I am certainly not suggesting that eating nuts will kill people, my point is that they contain toxins, many of which we have not yet identified or studied, and for which the long-term effects of ingestion are unknown.

Some of what we commonly refer to as nuts are also sometimes classified as fruits. One example is the almond, which in its wild form contains the glycoside amygdalin, which becomes transformed into deadly prussic acid (hydrogen cyanide) after crushing, chewing, or any other injury to the seed. The only way wild almonds could have been eaten was if they were processed by leaching or roasting to remove their toxicity, so they clearly were not a popular food of either PA or the chimpanzee. Selective breeding resulted in today's domesticated almond, but it is unknown and uncontrolled as to the remaining toxins or their concentration.

Cashews are a classical example of the nightmare of terminology in the botanical world. What appears to be the fruit of the cashew tree is an oval shaped *pseudo-fruit* called the cashew apple. It ripens into a yellow and/or red structure that is edible, and has a sweet smell and a sweet taste. What is referred to as the *true fruit* of the cashew tree is a kidney shaped hard shell within which is a single *seed*, called the cashew *nut*. The hard double shell contains a resin, urushiol, which is a potent skin irritant also found in botanically related poison ivy, leaving in doubt its use as an Ancient food.

What is the upside of eating nuts? They are a source of protein, but on the Original Diet, who needs more protein? They are supposedly a good source of minerals such as selenium, zinc, and magnesium, but paradoxically they contain anti-nutrients that bind minerals so that they are mostly unavailable. People have tried soaking and heating nuts to reduce the anti-effects sufficiently to make their mineral content available, but who knows. What we do know is that heating nuts damages the fragile polyunsaturated oils they contain (mostly omega-6), as does shelling them and leaving them exposed to light and air.

Brazil nuts are high in selenium, but as their name implies, they certainly were not native to Africa. Let's look at the Original Diet with respect to some of these minerals. Starting with selenium, research shows that the largest and most bioavailable proportion of human selenium intake is from meat, particularly beef. Plant forms of selenium are less available [98]. For zinc, research also shows that the largest and most bioavailable proportion of human zinc intake is from meat as opposed to plants [99]. With respect to magnesium, fresh fruit is a source, and contains no anti-nutrients to interfere with absorption.

The mineral water in the Original Diet adds significant minerals to the mix, including magnesium and calcium. This fact is often completely overlooked in the nutritional analyses of Paleo diets. As I stated above, applying nutrient RDA values to the PA diet makes little sense as they are based on the SAD diet, so the only benchmark we have for the Original Diet is 99,600 generations of accumulated data. I discuss the inadvisability of using nut and seed oils in a later section on cooking oils.

Coconut deserves some special consideration. The origins of the coconut, particularly in relation to Africa, are somewhat muddy, with conflicting opinions, including the claim that Polynesians brought them to Africa, or that they were indigenous to East Africa. The two closest botanical relatives to the coconut are found in southern Africa and Madagascar [100], which may have some bearing on early native African existence of coconut palms. Coconuts are not the easiest food to retrieve, but it is certainly doable by the nimble, and a large, sharp rock is sufficient to get at the goodies. Ripe coconuts are also known to drop on you unexpectedly. Unlike other nuts, coconut pulp and water, assuming it is not from a tree growing in polluted soil, has a very low toxin profile, but there have been some rare cases of people having allergic reactions to the pulp, and even the oil. Coconut water has actually been used intravenously as a rehydration fluid in emergencies [101].

As to why MA would leave the coconut more vulnerable than other nuts, my best guess is its size and tough shell, which makes it somewhat indestructible to all but clever humans late in the evolutionary history of palm trees. Having said all this, while its medium-chain fatty acid profile might be useful for people eating a SAD diet, I see no compelling nutritional reason to add coconut to the Original Diet. Small amounts could be tried as a snack if you are not sensitive to walnuts or almonds. As you are probably aware, tropical oils such as coconut and palm have been demonized because they are high in saturated vegetable fat, raising the heart-unhealthy arguments. From my research, this is nonsense, but I still do not encourage the use of any extracted oils in cooking.

For those non-purists who wish to eat some nuts, I would advise eating them raw, right out of the shell - there are many quality nutcrackers on the market. They should be stored in the refrigerator until shelled. Most nuts are rich in polyunsaturated oils, and out of their shells, the oils they contain can become readily rancid, since they are easily damaged by heat, air, and light. In their original natural packaging, the likelihood of damage is reduced. Of course, one still has the natural toxins to contend with, and raw nuts can be hard to digest (another clue from MA). Coconut, hazelnut, and macadamia nuts are low in phytates, and might make good choices for raw eating.

Roots, Stems and Leaves

It is interesting that most herbal medicinal preparations are derived from plant roots, stems, and leaves. What is going on here is that the toxins in these plant parts are being used medicinally to alleviate various symptoms. These are the same plant parts (including bark) that have been used by the pharmaceutical industry to derive drugs, all of which are also toxic. Why would you want to eat drugs as a regular part of your diet?

For those who wish to eat some vegetables, my best suggestion would be leaves or stems of very large plants such as trees. Presumably, MA would be less concerned about damage to a large plant from leaf or stem removal, and hence lessen the toxic load in these. There is some research to show that leaves in the upper reaches of trees have fewer toxins than those easily reachable, which makes sense as an evolutionary survival tactic [8]. There is every indication that the long neck of the giraffe evolved for the very purpose of reaching the less-toxic upper leaves of trees.

Remarkably, plants communicate with each other by giving off volatile compounds when under attack by a predator. Nearby plants react to the signal by quickly increasing the level of toxins they produce, in an attempt to ward off the predators. On the other hand, some animals have learned this trick, so they do not feed on adjacent plants, but move far enough away to find plants that did not get the warning signals. If only humans had not lost this intuition, perhaps we would be able to know the what, when, and how much answers as to which of the toxic parts of plants are safe to eat.

Sugars

Fruit is the main source of natural sugars in the Original Diet, and as previously indicated, I believe they should be eaten raw and not juiced. If sweet and edible, the skin has many nutrients as well as good fiber. The process of making sugar by evaporating juice from sugarcane first developed in India around 2,500 years ago. From there, sugar became a prized trading commodity, and eventually a huge cash crop throughout the world as a staple of cooking and dessert. The story of sugar refinement has been a horror story for humans, and along with it came dental caries, diabetes, and many other health problems. As far as artificial sweeteners are concerned, in my opinion (and those of others) they are all toxic, including the neurotoxins aspartame, and sucralose (a chlorine derivative) [102]. Strangely, from my research of the popular artificial sweeteners, saccharine is by far the least toxic. Stevia, a popular alternative sweetener, is derived from a leaf, hence not part of the Original Diet, and there have been some reports of its toxicity.

Honey, an insect product, is not on the Original Diet list for a few reasons. First, taking it from the hive interrupts the reproductive cycle of the bees (notwithstanding their considerable defenses), so I consider it doubtful MA would approve. Further, honey takes on the toxic properties of the flowers from which it was made, and there have been cases of life-threatening allergic and other toxic reactions as a result. Considering the fruit content of the Original Diet, there should be no need to supplement the diet with additional sugars. It is not rocket science that picking fruit it is a lot more fun than sticking a hand into a beehive, and the tropical African climate is conducive to year-round fruit availability.

Now for some potentially good news in the sweetener arena. Brazzein, a relatively new plant-based sweetener will soon be hitting the market [103]. Lo and behold, it is made from an African fruit! Assuming the sweetener is extracted from the fruit pulp or edible peel, as opposed to the seed, it should be an acceptable product in small quantities.

Extracted Oils

Extracted vegetable oils (from seeds) are a very recent addition to the SAD diet, and while they look clean and bright on the grocer's shelves, I cannot think of any reason to consume them. Of course, we have already eliminated seeds from the Original Diet, but I want to drive home the point with respect to seed oils so that there is no mistake as to my feelings on the subject.   I am referring to seed oils like safflower, sunflower, cottonseed, corn, sesame, peanut, walnut, pumpkin, canola, and the like. Oil processing begins with the extraction of crude vegetable oils from the seeds, a process that requires high temperatures and pressures, and sometimes involves a chemical solvent. Some of the steps involved in processing include caustic refining, bleaching, deodorizing, filtering, and removing saturates to make the oils more liquid. This has created a whole family of Frankenfats and dietary oils with unnatural molecular patterns, such as trans-fats, hydrogenated oils, cyclic fatty acid derivatives, cross-linked fatty acid chains, dimers, polymers, cross-linked triglycerides, and body-shifted molecules.

In the future, I expect we will uncover all kinds of additional molecular disturbances and toxic effects from oil that is heated. As one toxic byproduct after another is brought to the attention of the public (e.g. hydrogenated oils and trans-fats), in the vegetable oil industry, the lipid chemists go to work "eliminating" it, but from what I can see, they are merely creating others that for the moment remain hidden from the public eye. There is a lot of profit-driven creativity out there because these oils play a big role in the SAD diet.   For instance, scientists have apparently figured out how to heat a vegetable oil and not produce a measurable trans-fatty compound. They have engineered soybean and other vegetable oils into forms that can be heated all day. They test for trans-fats and there aren't any, but this is just another attempt to fool MA, and nobody knows the long-term effects.

For years, "Mediterranean diet" studies have made a nutritional celebrity out of olive oil. This oil is unique in that it is extracted from a fruit, the olive, as opposed to a seed, so perhaps it is a candidate for addition to the Original Diet. Well, the olive fruit straight from the tree is a very bitter one, and quite unpalatable raw unless processed in chemical solutions or fermented, so it does not qualify as a Original Diet fruit. Olive oil is high in oleic acid, a monounsaturated omega-9 fatty acid that our body does not need from foods, since it can make its own. So why has olive oil been singled out as very *healthy* (remember that this is a comparative term)? Well, when compared to the other oils sitting on the shelf, it is less unhealthy for the very reason that it is monounsaturated. Virtually all of the other oils are naturally high in omega-6 polyunsaturated fatty acids, which are more fragile and easily damaged by light, air, and heat, so many of them are rancid as they sit on the shelf. Therefore, olive oil wins by default, since omega-9 is more stable than omega-6 and, hence, less damaged by processing.

Canola oil (Canadian Oil) has become another favorite, thanks to a major marketing effort. It is made from a genetically modified form of rapeseed which, in its natural form, is toxic to humans and some animals [104]. Its fatty acid profile is similar to olive, and it contains some omega-3 fatty acids, which may well have been damaged by the many processing steps involved in production. A great deal of additional information on this oil can be found on the Weston Price Foundation website. Fortunately, no processed or extracted oils are needed in the Original Diet. I personally would not go near any of these oils, and would certainly not heat or otherwise cook with any poly- or monounsaturated oil. For anyone wanting to be a guinea pig and put their health in the hands of lipid chemists, the only oils that I could even suggest heating would be those high in saturated fats, such as coconut or palm oils, or animal fats such as beef, lamb and pork fat.

Liquids other than mineral/spring water

Liquids such as juices, teas, coffee, alcoholic beverages, sodas, sports drinks, dairy, and anything in a plastic or paper container are not a part of the Original Diet, with the following exceptions.

Fruit teas can be made by cutting and mashing some fresh fruit and adding it to hot water to make a drink. The so-called fruit teas on the market are not made with the fruit but are usually made with the leaves of the plant, which contain natural toxins. Examples are raspberry tea, which is actually made with raspberry leaf, not the fruit, and watermelon tea, which is actually made with watermelon seeds, not the fruit. I do not know of any commercial tea made with fruit pulp, but here is a way to make some that is somewhat easier than mashing fruit. One fruit farm, Brownwood Acres, produces a liquid fruit product that includes the acceptable parts of the fruit, namely the pulp and the skin. Presently, it is available using cherries, pomegranates, and a berry mix. This company identifies these products as liquid fruit supplements (as opposed to their concentrates, which are just the fruit juice) [105]. A teaspoon in hot water is plenty to make a fruit tea.

While I do not suggest it, fruit could be juiced using a slow speed, low temperature juicer, but the pulp should be put back into the glass. Also, the seeds or pits should be completely removed before juicing to avoid those toxins. Most commercial fruit juices are pasteurized, usually include additional sweeteners, and are devoid of the pulp.

This completes the discussion of the Tier Three food group. Before going on to the food preparation section, I would like to make a suggestion of how some of the Tier Three foods might be added to a Tier One/Two diet in a manner to moderate the impact they may have on the body defense system. Essentially, the idea would be to eat foods from only one subcategory on any one day. The subcategories are dairy, grains, beans, nuts, roots (and tubers), stems, leaves, sugars and extracted oils. My preference would be to avoid completely the sugar and extracted oil subcategories, and then choose foods from among the other seven subcategories on a rotation basis. For example, on one day add to the Tier One/Two foods some dairy food such as raw cheese, but no foods from any of the other Tier Three subcategories. On the next day, replace the dairy with some grain such as rice. On the next day, replace the grain with some nuts, and so on. The intent is to moderate the toxic load on the defense system by limiting the Tier Three subcategories to only one per day, and then rotate them. Perhaps a particular Tier Three subcategory would not be repeated more than once per week. While I have no evidence to back up my supposition regarding the moderating effect on the toxic load, I have to believe this approach will be an improvement over eating multiple Tier Three categories as a substantial part of the diet on a daily basis, which is the case with the SAD diet. To the extent you know you are allergic to or incompatible with a food subcategory, obviously avoid those foods.

Chapter 10 - Food Preparation

In this section, I will comment on various food preparation methods, and how they might, or might not, apply to the Original Diet. In general, I do not heat any of the fruit on the diet, but I do gently bake the meats that I eat, trying to keep them somewhat on the rare side.

Fermentation as practiced by humans is a relatively modern technique to try to make toxic plant foods and some dairy foods either less toxic or more nutritious. As stated previously, this sometimes backfires, and in the case of cruciferous vegetables such as cabbage, fermentation can actually increase the concentration of toxins. On the other hand, it is more than likely that PA would occasionally come across a piece of fermented fruit that had dropped from the parent plant, over-ripened and broken open, and been colonized by some yeast in the neighborhood, perhaps floating in the air. Some fermented fruit is known to have an alcohol content of ten percent or more, providing PA with an opportunity to become inebriated. Animals (and even insects) have been known to get totally wiped out on naturally fermented fruit, but it certainly has its disadvantages when there are predators hiding in the bushes. So, the supposition is that PA's binges would be few and far between, just based on survival instinct [8]. For the adventuresome reader, feel free to ferment a piece of allowable fruit on occasion. Let it not be said that you could not occasionally get buzzed on the Original Diet. Of course, wine is a fermented fruit (grapes), so I leave it to the reader regarding experimentation in this area. Note that for those with a Candida overgrowth problem (discussed in *The Wellness Project*) alcohol greatly aggravates this condition.

From a review of some of the modern hunter-gatherer societies such as the Inuit and the American Indian, as well as from studying the behavior of carnivorous animals, it is clear that the intestinal contents of herbivorous prey animals were also consumed. This would consist of fermented or partially fermented plant products such as grass for a ruminant like a buffalo, or plankton in the case of a seal [16], and would contain the valuable spore-forming bacteria discussed earlier. In our modern diet, it would be hard to come by this delicacy. The nearest commercial product I can think of is raw sauerkraut or Kim chi, but neither the vegetables used nor the fermenting medium match up with what we are after, and they contain natural toxins. So, out of a sense of frustration, I set about devising a way that we could reproduce healthy fermented food (see the side box entitled An Artificial Cow Gut).

An Artificial Cow Gut

In an effort to mass-produce the fermented intestinal contents of, say, a cow, I proposed the following. In a suitably heated container (heated to the temperature of a functioning cow gut), mix together the typical natural foods of a cow (grass, clover, etc.) with the bacteria and enzymes normally found in a healthy cow gut, which were extracted in a humane manner. Stir and heat until fermentation takes place in the container, then remove a portion for consumption. Add more grass to continue the process indefinitely. Wouldn't it be great to turn the grass from your newly mowed (chemical free) lawn into a dinner side dish? I have filed a patent application covering the making of this food using this method, in the hope that it will interest a forward-thinking food producer to give it a try.

Until the actual cow gut contents or a synthesized version become available, very small amounts of raw (unpasteurized) sauerkraut might be ingested on occasion, with the caveat that it contains thyroid hormone disrupters. Spore forming bacteria supplements can also be used to supplement the diet, which will at least represent a portion of the bacterial component of animal gut contents. The interesting thing about this component of the Original Diet is that it brings vegetables into it, but in a form that nature intended, that is, preprocessed by the gut of an herbivore that Nature designed to eat the stuff.

Previously, I stated that I bake my animal foods but try to keep the cooking time and temperature to a minimum because heat damages food, and the more you heat, the more you damage. Pasteurization is a classical example. At the far extreme is frying, which is cooking food surrounded by a fat or oil that is heated to a very high temperature. We have already discussed the dangers of heating fats or oils other than those that are mainly saturated, because their chemical structure resists heat damage better than the unsaturates. I do not believe PA would have been using frying to cook animal products. The lowest temperature method of cooking meat would be boiling it in water, which ensures that no portion of the meat exceeds the boiling point of water. Archeological evidence seems to point to the use of hearth-like structures that may have been used to indirectly heat the food, say, by using a bed of clay or one or more heated rocks in a manner similar to baking, which is the method I use. I prefer electric heat as opposed to gas, because of the potentially toxic byproducts of burning gas, and the likelihood that they will be absorbed into the food. A convection-type oven works well, eliminates oven hot spots, and speeds up the cooking process. An example of an inexpensive counter-top convection oven is widely sold under the Aroma Housewares Aeromatic brand.

I do not use microwave cooking. The debate on the dangers of microwaving food has been going on for years, but independent research is limited. Who's going to pay to study it? Certainly not the microwave industry, which ranges from the device manufacturers themselves to the companies that produce instant, microwavable food. There is no real money in proving that microwaves are toxic. A few studies have been done and they tend to be negative enough for me, so for that reason, I don't use a microwave [106]. In particular, one study showed that microwave heating converts the amino acid l-proline to d-proline. They write, "The conversion of *trans* to *cis* forms could be hazardous because when *cis*-amino acids are incorporated into peptides and proteins instead of their *trans* isomers, this can lead to structural, functional and immunological changes." They further note that "d-proline is neurotoxic and we have reported nephrotoxic and heptatotoxic effects of this compound" [107]. Proline is found in large quantities in gelatin, an integral part of animal foods. So, one can assume that when animal foods are heated in the microwave, they may become toxic to the liver, kidneys and nervous system.

It is now well-recognized that microwaving food in plastic containers is a very bad idea because the heated plastic (and other materials) can outgas toxic substances into the food [108]. Even the use of so-called microwavable plastics is not part of an experiment I want to participate in because we have yet to identify all of the toxins in the various plastics, let alone the safe levels of each, if there are any.

As far as cooking utensils go, I cook in glass dishes and do not let the food come in contact with metal racks, some of which are chrome or nickel-plated and may tend to flake off. Even stainless steel is not impervious to outgassing, and it contains chromium and nickel, both toxic in large quantities. Aluminum is a neurotoxin, so I avoid any aluminum-containing cookware, and I also avoid coated products, even porcelain. Their bright colors are provided by metal pigments of unknown origin. Teflon-coated cookware has been in the news of late because when heated, some of the compounds in Teflon become extremely toxic and potentially carcinogenic.

Uncolored glass is the way to go for me, and brands such as Pyrex® are inexpensive and come in every possible shape you might need, some with handles. I cook with Pyrex and use it for storage; it is available with plastic tops but they do not come in direct contact with the food. The beauty of glass is that you can take it right out of the refrigerator, cook it in the same container, and know it is safe.

For serving pieces, I opt for uncolored glass or ceramic. For silverware, my suggestion is real silver, not stainless. The ideal is sterling silver, which is an alloy of silver and very small amounts of a metal such as copper, zinc or platinum. Yes, you may take out the "special-occasion-only" sterling flatware and use it every day – aren't you entitled to it? Silver is a somewhat unique heavy metal in its interactions with the body. It has antibacterial, antifungal, and antiviral properties, yet in very small quantities it does not appear to have toxic effects. In large quantities, it can discolor the skin gray (argyria) somewhat permanently and can be neurotoxic. I do not foresee a problem using silver as flatware, but I would not cook in it or use it for hot drink containers. Modernly, silver is available in colloidal form and as nanoparticles for use as a supplement. It is gaining wide acceptance in the medical instrument field as a coating, and is also available in bandages for its antiseptic properties. Silver plate is another option for flatware, but a concern is that the plate will either wear or chip off, exposing the base metal.

Chapter 11 - Food Supplements

You might wonder how I can make a pitch for supplements when I'm advocating a natural, prehistoric type of diet? Unfortunately, for a variety of reasons, it is somewhat impossible to reproduce nutritionally in its entirety the Original Diet or even some of the other indigenous diets. One reason is that some of the foods are simply not available, such as a hippo, or a mammoth, or some of the exotic African fruits. Another reason is that, even if available, we have not developed a taste for some of the important animal parts such as the various organs, blood and marrow, or there is fear of human-made contamination. Yet another reason, particularly in the fruit category, is that modern cultivation practices are yielding produce that is estimated to have significantly reduced nutritional profiles (vitamins and minerals) as compared to their ancient wild-grown counterparts, even those that are organically grown. As the name implies, mineral water is a major source of minerals, particularly calcium and magnesium, and we know from studies that people living near and using mountain stream water tend to live longer, healthier lives. So it behooves us to insure that the mineral water we are drinking is accompanied by high levels of these important minerals.

In the 21st century, one has to be creative and practical in order to fill in the missing ingredients and round out Nature's diet as best as possible. The following supplements help to do that, but please bear in mind that most food supplements are human-made or in some way tampered with so that they no longer have a counterpart in nature, no matter what the marketing folks would like you to believe. Therefore, these supplements have the potential of being toxic. One simple example is that virtually all capsule and tablet products use stearic acid or magnesium stearate as an added ingredient to speed up packaging. Theoretically, these ingredients can be sourced from seed oils, and perhaps even be hydrogenated. Fortunately, on the Original Diet, only a very few supplements are even suggested, and many of them are natural. As far as those folks on other diets such as the SAD diet, enormous amounts of supplements may be necessary just to keep them going.

As you recall from the dirt section of the diet, supplements to supply fulvic/humic acids as well as spore-forming bacteria were discussed. Because I consider them an intimate part of the diet itself, they are not repeated here.

Vitamins

I have found that, until a certain amount of detoxification has taken place, taking large doses of vitamins as supplements can be very counterproductive because they feed the bad guys. As an example, the yeast Candida loves many of the B-vitamins, and taking large doses can easily contribute to its overgrowth. Actually, some B vitamins are normally produced for us by the microflora in our intestines, such as vitamin B6 [109], but many of us have disturbed gut flora due to toxins, so supplements can be helpful. If we look to MA for guidance, we find that another major source of B-vitamins for PA would have been the liver of prey animals, probably eaten raw. Most liver lovers like to eat it fried, and the attendant high cooking temperatures may destroy much of the vitamin content. Another modern concern in eating liver is its potential toxicity.

Many people, including myself, have assumed that taking a B-vitamin supplement can provide us with the equivalent of what is missing from our food sources. It was not until I did some serious research into the nutritional advantages of liver that I discovered many animal studies that showed this is not necessarily true. Dating back to the 1950's, Benjamin Ershoff, a medical researcher, ran dozens of experiments with rats to determine the effects of various nutritive substances on the health of the animals when they are subjected to various toxins and other stressors. In several of these experiments he tested the use of B- vitamin supplements versus small amounts of raw desiccated (dried) liver added to the diets of the rats, who were then subjected to various stressors such as swimming, x-ray radiation, thyroid hormone disrupters and the like [110, 111]. In each instance, he found that the rats fed liver outperformed and out-survived those fed synthetic B- vitamins. His conclusion was there is something in liver that we are unaware of that provides benefits beyond just B-vitamin supplementation. I don't know of any studies directed to finding out what these substances might be. We do know that the liver is the major detoxification organ, and perhaps some of these detox agents remain in raw liver and provide a protective effect.

Armed with this information, I set about looking at the various raw liver supplements on the market to see if any would be a suitable addition to the diet. My criteria were that it had to be derived from organic grass-fed animals in a protected environment to avoid toxins, and it had to be processed using low-temperatures to avoid damaging the tissue components. A final criterion was that the supplement should include both the water-soluble and fat-soluble portions of the liver, because Ershoff found that the combination was an important factor in its efficacy. Several desiccated beef liver supplements are available that are made from protected Argentinean free-range grass fed beef, and they use low temperature processing. However, I could only find one that was not defatted. It is supplied by Now Foods as a powder or a tablet [112], and is the product I use as a basic B- vitamin supplement. I happen to like the taste of liver, so I chew five tablets at each meal, or put one teaspoon of the powder in my fruit tea. For those who do not like the taste, swallowing the tablets is the way to go. Because this supplement is really a food, you can munch on it during the day for an energy boost. There is a long history of bodybuilders downing fistfuls of liver tablets for stamina.

Before leaving the subject of B- vitamins, I want to single out what I (and others) consider the queen of this group, and that is vitamin B6. It is responsible for more enzyme reactions in the body than any of the other vitamins, and its proper assimilation is easily interfered with by a variety of toxins, including candida overgrowth. I consider its supplementation to be important in conjunction with the modern implementation of the Original Diet for the following reason. There is some evidence that today's cultivated fruit is higher in sugars than the wild counterparts available to PA [46]. Studies have also shown that consumption of sugars has the effect of depleting vitamin B6 in the body [113] [114]. High levels of vitamin B6 are found in fruit as well as liver, important foods in the Original Diet. However, the importance of vitamin

B6 to so many of the body's processes, coupled with a higher sugar intake from modern cultivated fruits leads me to add a daily vitamin B6 supplement to my regimen as a precautionary factor. It is usually found in supplement form as pyridoxine HCl, which must be converted in the body to the active form, pyridoxal–5'-phosphate (P5P). Because some toxins, including Candida overgrowth, can interfere with this conversion, I take P5P directly. Further, because P5P is easily damaged by stomach acid, I take it in the form of a sublingual tablet, placed under the tongue to dissolve and directly enter the bloodstream. The one I use, at four tablets per day, is Coenzymated B-6, made by Source Naturals [115].

Vitamin C is in the news almost daily as either being a panacea for major illnesses or being demonized for one thing or another. First, we need some definitions. Vitamin C is found in plant and animal products. In animals, it appears to be in the form of pure ascorbic acid, and this is the form usually called Vitamin C. In plants, primarily fruits and leaves, it is also found in the form of ascorbic acid, but it is virtually always found along with a group of compounds called bioflavonoids which I will call the "flavonoid complex". In the animal world, all mammals except for a small group including primates, humans, guinea pigs, the red-vented bulbul (a fruit-eating bird), a species of trout, and the Indian fruit bat can make their own vitamin C. This group apparently lost the ability to do so, supposedly because ample amounts were provided in their diet. Can we find some clues from MA as to what is going on?

Well, starting with fruit bats and the bulbul, they are major fruit eaters, eating the sweet stuff and spitting out the seeds as part of MA's plan to further plant germination. In the plant world, fruit, second only to some leaves, is the major source of vitamin C. Guinea pigs are not pigs, but rodents native to South America. There is precious little information available about their native diet because they have become so domesticated. There is even some discussion that they are now rarely found in the wild (they are a favorite food in many South American countries). Apparently, they like to eat grass, but so do many other rodents as well as rabbits, so I remain clueless as to why the guinea pig was singled out to lose the capacity to make vitamin C.

Primates eat a lot of fruit and leaves, so they should have a large intake of vitamin C. In one study, it was estimated that monkeys weighing about 15 pounds had an average daily intake of about 700 mg of vitamin C, while gorillas weighing 200-300 pounds had daily intakes in the 2-4 gram region [46]. I estimate a desirable human vitamin C intake in the range of 0.5-3 grams on the Original Diet. As you will see from the discussion below, Vitamin C needs can vary widely with stress level.

There is a lot more to the vitamin C puzzle than just my short analysis, and I have experimented with some enormous doses over the years, both orally and intravenously, while on the Original Diet. I can't say I received any particular beneficial or adverse effects (except diarrhea on high oral doses), even up to occasional 50 gram IV doses, but then again, I have not had a cold or even a sniffle while on the Original Diet. I do know that in general the human bowel tolerance for vitamin C changes drastically upward when the body is under stress. This takes us to another part of the puzzle: the observation that animals that produce their own vitamin C supply also have a built-in control system that increases the amount produced (sometimes up to several hundred grams) in response to stress, which we, of course, cannot mimic without taking supplements.

This animal behavior has led me to speculate as follows: let us say a band of PA hunters is in the chase to take down an African buffalo, and the buffalo knows it. Presumable, this is a high-stress situation for the buffalo, and consequently hundreds of grams of vitamin C are being produced and pumped throughout the animal's body. If so, when caught and eaten, perhaps PA was taking in from the meat somewhat massive amounts of vitamin C, information that I have not seen considered in past dietary studies. I don't have an answer, but we do know that PA favored glands and other organs from prey, and we also know that the adrenal glands usually contain the highest concentrations of vitamin C, so this is another source.

Since we and this small group of other mammals have lost not only the ability to make vitamin C, but also the ability to generate large amounts during stress, this leads me to another two-part theory as to why MA cut us off. First, we get enough from our diet, and second, we have evolved as low-stress animals (as compared to the rest of the mammal world), and hence not in need of the vitamin C stress-enhancement capability. I bring up this point again in the magnesium and chronic stress discussions below. I do not know of any studies in this area, but it would be a fun research project.

Regarding vitamin C (ascorbic acid) supplementation, many of the products on the market are derived from corn, most of which is GMO (Genetically Modified Organism). Some corn-free products that are available are derived from cassava root (also called tapioca), or sago palm, all of which appear to be synthetically derived. I use corn-free Vitamin C 500 mg by Nature's Plus. I take one ascorbic acid cap with each meal.

Regarding Vitamin E, the very term is ill defined. It generally refers to alpha-tocopherol, which is found in nature only as part of a complex of tocopherols and tocotrienols. I try to avoid supplements that contain alpha-tocopherol as an isolated nutrient, since it is not found in nature that way and there is now some evidence that it may prove toxic in its isolated form. A better choice is a vitamin E complex supplement that contains several E components, including both tocopherols and tocotrienols. There are several such E-complexes on the market, and the starting material for many is red palm oil (see for example U.S. Patent 5,157,132). This oil is extracted from the fruit of the oil palm, which, lo and behold, is an Original Diet food, having passed the ABC test. So instead of messing with the supplement products, one would ideally eat oil palm fruit, which is described as somewhat fibrous and oily. However, I am not aware of any readily available sources for the fruit. Instead, I suggest chugalugging some red palm oil (not palm kernel oil, which is derived from the nut), which is extracted from the fruit and which is readily available. Not only is it high in the E complex, it is also very high in the pro-vitamin A carotenoid complex, and in vitamin K.

Just as alpha-tocopherol is not found in nature as an isolate, beta-carotene is similarly not found that way, and I try to avoid any supplements that contain beta-carotene as an isolated ingredient. Some studies have shown that beta-carotene may be toxic in isolated form, particularly when Candida overgrowth may be present. Red palm oil contains the carotenoid complex as found in nature, which includes alpha, beta, and other carotenoids yet to be defined. From my studies, red palm oil has the highest edible concentrations of Vitamin E and carotenoid complexes in the plant kingdom. Red palm oil is also high in vitamin K1, useful in controlling blood clotting, and as a raw material for enzyme processes in your body that helps keep calcium out of your arterial walls and bring it into your bones.

An interesting property of vitamins pro-A, E and K is that their absorption is increased significantly when consumed with fat, which is amply provided in the palm oil itself, as well as in the rest of the Original Diet. I take one to three teaspoons of the oil per day, right off the spoon. The kind I look for is Organic Virgin Palm Oil, which is red in color, originates in Africa, and is not refined, deodorized, or bleached. One source is Tropical Traditions [116]. Red palm oil has been demonized as unhealthy because it is high in saturated fat, a red herring for heart disease [117]. For those who want to forgo taking red palm oil directly, a trio of supplements would be needed just to replace the pro-A, E and K components. Some suggestions would be CarotenAll by Jarrow [118], and *Super K* and *Gamma E Tocopherol/Tocotrienols*, both from Life Extension Foundation [119].

Vitamin D is another critical nutrient, and acts both as a vitamin and as a prohormone. The ideal natural source is from the UVB spectrum of ultraviolet light impinging on unprotected skin, and I feel confident that PA had no shortage of sunlight in the tropics. I already commented above on my theory regarding skin cancer, and I go into more depth on this subject in the lifestyle section. Modernly, unless you happen to live in a tropical or semi-tropical environment, it is quite difficult for people in Western societies to get sufficient sunlight year round to produce adequate vitamin-D, which has been found to be necessary for bone strength and it is a potent anti-cancer compound [120]. Alternatives to getting natural sunlight include an artificial UVB source using a UV bulb (discussed in the lifestyle section); obtaining vitamin-D from the diet (liver is a source); and obtaining vitamin-D from supplements. Serious research into Vitamin-D is just beginning, and there is much that remains unknown, including all of the various forms that make up what will undoubtedly become the "Vitamin-D complex" some time in the future. Because we don't know yet what we are doing in this area, the best course of action is to follow MA, and get it from UV.

I personally prefer a UVB lamp, but supplements are an alternative. Before taking any, I suggest getting a Vitamin-D blood test. The test is called 25(OH)D, or 25-hydroxyvitamin D, and the latest consensus seems to be that an optimum level is above 30 and below 60 ng/ml. Excessively low or high levels can be harmful. If the level is low, Vitamin-D3 supplements are available (avoid Vitamin-D2 since it is poorly absorbed and interferes with magnesium absorption). One source I have used is Biotics Research Bio-D-Mulsion (available in 400 IU and 2000IU drops). Getting to the right dose (say between 1200 and 8000 IU per day) requires experimentation and monitoring using the 25(OH)D test [121].

As is the case in so many of the tests designed to measure levels of various compounds in the body, the vitamin D test results have generated confusion. A study was conducted where the 25(OH)D test was run on a group of people in Honolulu who habitually obtained a great amount of sun exposure. It was found that 51% of the tested group had a test level below the 30 ng/ml lower cutoff, indicating vitamin D deficiency [122]. This leaves for speculation whether the test is unreliable or a large subset of the population does not properly produce vitamin D, even with significant UVB exposure. Until this discrepancy can be sorted out, I continue to prefer UVB exposure as the natural way to obtain vitamin D, on the basis that at least MA knows what she is doing.

Regarding the relationship between UV and melanoma, the most deadly form of skin cancer, there are about as many studies showing incidence increase with excessive sun exposure as those that show the opposite [123] [124]. Something I find puzzling in these studies is that it did not strike the researchers that those people who sunburn easily might also be those with a compromised defense system, making them more susceptible to cancer, independent of sun exposure. At lease empirically, it is well- known that, for example, deranged fatty acid synthesis (typical of eating the SAD diet) can cause a person to be very susceptible to sunburning as opposed to tanning.

Minerals - The Magnesium Factor

The title of this section is borrowed from a very important book of the same name, *The Magnesium Factor*, by Mildred Seelig, MD [25]. As you will see, magnesium, of all of the essential minerals, is not only the most overlooked and most deficient, but in my opinion, is also the most critical to our health. I will start with mineral supplementation in general, then move on to magnesium and finally to some of the support nutrients that work together to ensure an adequate supply of this critical nutrient.

Concerning minerals and the Original Diet, it would appear that PA derived certain of her/his minerals from two sources. The first is from food sources such as animal parts and fruit, and the second source is mineral water. Accordingly, I have divided mineral supplementation into two sections, one taken with food, and the other taken with water.

For food-based mineral supplementation, I take a multi-mineral to bolster what might be deficient in modern animal and fruit products. My preference is a supplement without copper (usually already elevated as a result of many toxins including Candida), and without iron (there is no shortage of iron in meat), and one where the minerals are bound to fruit acids. Examples of fruit-acid-derived compounds are citrates, fumarates, malates, and succinates. I also like a high magnesium/calcium ratio because of the importance of magnesium, discussed further below. There is no ideal mineral supplement, and they all contain human-made ingredients of one sort or another. I use *Citramin II* by Thorne Research [68], which is based on citric acid and is iron and copper free. I take three per day with meals.

For water-based mineral supplementation, the macrominerals calcium and magnesium appear in large quantities in natural mountain spring water. As you know from my discussion of water, I go to great lengths to ensure a high mineral content in drinking water. The water mineral content is dependent upon municipal water sources, which vary greatly, and the use of RO and distillation filters depletes water of these vital nutrients. One solution, mentioned above, is to supplement drinking water with small amounts of dolomite, which provide calcium and magnesium in the natural ratio of approximately 1.7 to 1. A protocol I have used is one dolomite tablet with water up to four times per day, for a maximum of four tablets. See the digestive rehabilitation section for more information regarding dolomite and stomach acid.

While we are on the subject of dolomite, as mentioned earlier, the minerals that are present in mineral water are in the form of bicarbonates, while the minerals in dolomite are in the form of carbonates. If we want to match exactly the bicarbonate form as a supplement, this can be done with some effort. Basically, mixing dolomite powder with carbonated water will do the trick. I have certainly experimented with this method, and have concluded that the carbonate form as found in dolomite not only has a long history of successful use, but works as well for me as the bicarbonate form. From a chemistry perspective, both the bicarbonate and carbonate mineral forms are expected to dissociate into chlorides in the body in the presence of stomach acid

Under "normal" circumstances, what I just described would appear to provide sufficient mineral supplementation, but we do not live under normal circumstances. Most of us live in a high chronic stress environment that has a major impact on depleting our body stores of magnesium, which I regard as the most important of all of the essential minerals. As you shall see from the following, I pay a great deal of attention to ensuring adequate levels of this mineral.

For this discussion of magnesium, I will be drawing upon the excellent research in Dr. Seelig's book [25], as well as the book *The Miracle of Magnesium* by Carolyn Dean, MD [26], and others. It is well recognized that those on the SAD diet have a deficient intake of magnesium from all of the processed foods being eaten. Further, as already mentioned, many of the seed- and nut-based foods in that diet contain natural mineral-binding toxins such as phytates and oxalates that block the uptake of magnesium as well as other minerals. On the Original Diet, we have eliminated the processed foods and the mineral-binders, and we get lots of magnesium from the water and fruit portions of the diet alone, so magnesium intake should not normally be a problem. In spite of this, we may end up with a magnesium deficiency because of our modern lifestyle. It turns out that *stress* depletes magnesium in great quantities from our bodies, so that amounts that were sufficient for PA are not sufficient for us with our chronically stressful modern lifestyles.

Readers may take exception to the conclusion that PA did not lead a chronically stressful life, but the studies of modern hunter-gatherers, such as those in Weston Price's research, show people who, for the most part, are happy, peaceful, and content with their lives. As previously mentioned, the fact that we do not make our own vitamin C tends toward the conclusion that, from an evolutionary perspective, our ancestor's lives were substantially less chronically stressful than our present lifestyle. I have no doubt that PA experienced times of acute (meaning short term) episodes of stress during hunting and predator evasion, but that is quite different from chronic stress that hangs around 24/7 in our modern environment.

Much has been written about the detrimental effects of chronic stress on our health, but there is little to pinpoint the relationship. Some believe that the increased levels of adrenaline and cortisol produced by the adrenal glands in response to stress contribute to illness, and then there is an entire "industry" devoted to the treatment of adrenal fatigue, which may well turn out to be the result of magnesium deficiency, usually in combination with a toxin overload. I can remember puzzling over the mind/body connection in relation to physical health for many years. How does stress make one sick? Well, Dr. Seelig maps it out very clearly. Everyday stressors that we take for granted, such as loud noises, reading the newspaper, listening to the news, politics, or even driving on the freeway cause our bodies to excrete large amounts of magnesium, which is needed for more than 300 critically important chemical reactions in our body. Physical stressors as simple as working in the heat or jogging use up or excrete large amounts of magnesium, as does exposure to toxins.

Magnesium deficiency can show up in many ways. Let's start with the one that first caught my attention: sudden death. I presume many of you can remember young, excellent athletes at the peak of health that suddenly drop dead when jogging. How about the patient that drops dead while on the treadmill in the doctor's office. Or the elderly gentleman who, in a fit of anger over some issue, grabs his chest and keels over. From my research, magnesium is the key to these disasters, and this is just the tip of the iceberg.

The above scenarios relate to the role of magnesium as a muscle relaxant, where it works in opposition to calcium, which causes muscles to contract. Some early signs of magnesium-related neuromuscular symptoms as a result of depletion include twitching, muscle cramps anywhere, including finger, toe, wrist, and back, heel and other bone pain, difficulty swallowing, headaches, tinnitus and hearing loss, spastic gut functions including reflux, and heart fibrillations. Further compounding the issue is the fact that magnesium interacts with other minerals, whereby a deficiency of magnesium can cause a deficiency of potassium [125], as well as zinc, and an over-abundance of calcium can interfere with magnesium absorption. Additionally, magnesium and vitamin B-6 assist each other in absorption, and the assimilation of this vitamin is, in turn, impaired by a variety of toxins.

A second major category of symptoms from magnesium depletion relates to its role in the production of energy. It is a critical factor in the production of ATP (adenosine triphosphate), which can be thought of as the body's batteries. Therefore, a deficiency of magnesium can result in serious fatigue and low exercise stamina. It is also thought by many to be a cause of Chronic Fatigue Syndrome. Now here is the Catch-22 with respect to fatigue. Many of the usual remedies to alleviate fatigue involve increasing the metabolism or energy state of the body, all of which require magnesium to do their job, further depleting the body's reserves and actually aggravating the fatigue.

Speaking of the body's reserves, much of the magnesium is found in the bones and muscles, so depletion can result in fragile bones and weak muscles. Depletion can also result in high cholesterol levels, and interference with essential fatty acid processing by the body. Magnesium deficiency is also implicated in kidney and gall stones, prostate problems, hyper-excitability, asthma, ulcers, depression, suicidal impulses, pituitary malfunction, and even body odor [52] [126] [127]. There are also studies that show magnesium supplementation halts the progression of polio if used early enough. By now, you probably get my drift that we are talking about a seriously important nutrient. A great deal of research on the effects of magnesium deficiency on the body can be found at several websites [49, 128]. Because it is involved in so many enzyme reactions in the body, the list of deficiency symptoms is very extensive.

I can personally tell you that if magnesium is depleted, many of the food supplements and detoxification remedies discussed here will not work and can produce adverse results. My analysis of this is that many of them require magnesium in particular to perform their functions, so they draw from an already depleted supply, thus increasing the depletion problem and leading to more symptoms. One example is the attempt to treat adrenal fatigue. It turns out that the typical remedies of hydrocortisone, DHEA, licorice, and thyroid hormone all deplete magnesium, and to some extent potassium, so it is quite important to achieve proper mineral levels before trying any of these remedies.

Magnesium replenishment is not so easy. The established approach for nutrient supplementation is to test for a deficiency and if there is one, to supplement to restore the level. For magnesium, there are challenges both to testing the body's level and to supplementation. For example, routine blood tests ordered by the majority of doctors do not test for magnesium. The standard chemistry panel only tests for three of the four body electrolytes (sodium, potassium, and calcium), leaving out magnesium, an incredibly important mineral. One reason is that a serum blood test for magnesium is virtually useless because magnesium is primarily stored in the cells. A more meaningful test would be a magnesium red blood cell test, which is a special lab order (meaning it costs more money), and even it is not extremely accurate [129]. A test that has been found to be more accurate in measuring all of the electrolytes is known as the EXATEST by Intracellular Diagnostics, Inc., and it may be covered by insurance [130]. This test uses cells scraped from the floor of the mouth to make the evaluation. Based on the test results, a supplementation program can begin.

Regarding magnesium supplementation, a problem with using oral supplements is a tendency toward creating diarrhea at the high doses that may be necessary to restore proper body levels. One method of finding the maximum tolerable oral dose is to increase it slowly until loose stools occur, then back off to a point where the stool is normal, referred to as the bowel tolerance point. Diarrhea should not be prolonged because it will flush most minerals out of the body, as well as cause dehydration.

Slow-release magnesium compounds have been developed in an effort to address the diarrhea problem, but the unknown with any timed-release or sustained–release product is how much is actually being absorbed in the gut. It is very much dependent upon the individual's gut environment, not exactly a controlled variable. One approach to oral magnesium supplementation is simply to ingest more magnesium carbonate, the form of magnesium found in dolomite. It is available as Magnesium Carbonate in 135 mg tablets from BodyBio [131].

There are many other choices for oral magnesium supplementation. Many of them combine the metal with either a fruit acid, such as citrates and malates, or an amino acid, such as glycine. A particularly serendipitous combination is magnesium and the amino acid taurine, which form magnesium taurate. Taurine actually exhibits some of the same properties as magnesium, and they complement each other in the body [132]. Further, taurine can be of great use in alleviating the symptoms of Candida overgrowth. One brand of Magnesium Taurate capsules is by Cardiovascular Research/Ecological Formulas, widely available with 125 mg of magnesium per capsule. Another brand is Magnesium Taurate tablets by Douglas Labs, with 200 mg of magnesium per tablet [133].

I use either the carbonate or the taurate form in conjunction with the dolomite protocol. Daily magnesium dosages required to sustain normal body levels can vary widely from, say, 400 mg to 2 grams, and may be a function of one's toxin level (including chronic stress), among other things. For example, if you have high levels of lead, which accumulates in the bones, it may take larger amounts of magnesium to displace and replace the lead in the bone matrix (more on this in *The Wellness Project*).

Here are the oral magnesium supplement protocols that I have used in an effort to prevent diarrhea and assimilate large amounts of magnesium. I start with dolomite, and add additional magnesium as either magnesium carbonate or taurate or some of both. On an individual basis as part of the various detox protocols, and depending upon the toxin types and degree of toxicity being addressed, I would expect that daily doses of the various ingredients could typically range up to 4 dolomite tablets (containing 630 mg calcium and 350 mg magnesium) with 200-800 mg of additional magnesium. The dolomite tends toward constipation, and the magnesium has a laxative effect, so the objective is to balance the two to achieve normal stools and high magnesium intake. Taurine acts to stimulate the production of stomach acid, which assists in the assimilation of the dolomite.

Remarkably, even the above oral supplement protocol may not be sufficient to restore magnesium levels, or may take a long time to do so. One way to increase magnesium levels more quickly without causing diarrhea is to use a topical application. An established protocol is the use of magnesium sulphate crystals, known as Epsom salts, in bath water, which is quite soothing to some. Another protocol, and the one that I favor, is to wipe or spray on the skin a magnesium chloride solution -

several such products are available. One that I use is Dr. Shealy's Biogenics Magnesium Lotion [134]. Apply an amount equivalent to about two teaspoons twice a day to random skin areas and either leave it on or wash it off after 20 minutes. You can also obtain from this same source magnesium chloride crystals for use in a foot or body bath. I believe the chloride portion of magnesium chloride will also assist in displacing toxic halides such as bromide from the body.

I regard the topical application of magnesium as a very important adjunct protocol to aid in the restoration and maintenance of magnesium, and I plan to use it on a continuous basis. Dr. Shealy, a pioneer in the use of topically applied magnesium, estimates that it may take from 6 to 12 months to restore magnesium levels to normal using oral supplements [135]. For topical application, using the dosage listed above, he found that restoration occurred in 4 weeks. I apply the magnesium lotion twice daily, and I use a footbath several times per week with four ounces of the magnesium chloride crystals.

Still another approach to rapid magnesium replenishment is IV administration, as a slow drip of vitamins and minerals in what is known as a Myer's Cocktail [136], which usually includes magnesium sulphate. There are many variations of this cocktail, and the one I favor contains at least one gram of magnesium chloride. Ten drips may be sufficient to restore levels. Overdosing of magnesium is an unlikely occurrence unless a person has impaired kidney function, since excesses are readily excreted.

As it turns out, saturated fat in the diet interferes with the absorption of oral magnesium supplements. The theory is that magnesium binds with the fat in the gut to form insoluble salts, unusable by the body. Looking at PA's diet, where much of the magnesium was likely supplied by mineral-rich water, it is likely that a portion of his/her intake of magnesium occurred between meals, away from fat intake. So I take some of my magnesium and other mineral supplements with my water away from meals.

I am now going to go out on another limb (aren't trees handy) and speculate that this saturated fat/magnesium interaction may be a very important factor that has led to the incorrect demonizing of saturated fats. Let's begin with the proven fact that on the SAD diet in this modernly stressful world, most people are already marginally or very deficient in magnesium [25]. Even a slight increase in saturated fat in the diet could reduce the already deficient magnesium levels even further by binding up a portion of whatever magnesium is available, leading to a cascade of cardiovascular issues.

First, cholesterol levels may rise, leading to the incorrect conclusion that saturated fats are the cause of elevated cholesterol. Second, magnesium depletion is well known to lead to arterial plaque formation, hypertension, and virtually every other major sign of heart disease [25]. If my supposition is correct, this is yet another example of the medical community coming to the wrong conclusion regarding cause and effect relationships. My hypothesis seems to fit the fact pattern that some people can eat saturated fat and not have cardiovascular issues. It would be of great interest to measure their magnesium levels. I would guess that these folks have sufficient magnesium, while those that exhibit heart problems have a deficiency. It also explains why there is poor correlation between one's lipid profile and heart disease.

A lipid profile is actually an indirect reflection of body magnesium level, because there is not a consistent correlation between cholesterol level and magnesium level, just an inverse relationship. This is yet another example of measuring something indirectly that can be easily measured directly, assuming you know what to look for. What is needed is a study directly comparing magnesium level with CVD (Cardiovascular Disease), but there is no money in proving that magnesium supplementation is the correct treatment for CVD. What might really scare off statin-industry-paid researchers is that magnesium has the potential of reducing cholesterol in exactly the same way as do statin drugs, but without any side effects [28]. When you consider that virtually nobody in the medical field even bothers to measure body magnesium levels, you end up with the potential for a serious amount of faulty research being published. Because magnesium is *the* heart nutrient, at a minimum the magnesium levels of all participants in any cardiovascular study should be measured and published. This is not rocket science.

Now, let's look at some of the cofactor nutrients that work with magnesium. Our friend vitamin B6, previously discussed, is an important cofactor that aids in magnesium (and calcium) absorption in the body and is interfered with by many toxins, more reason to add it to the supplement list [137] [138].

Zinc is another mineral that appears to be depleted by many toxins, and it also requires sufficient body magnesium levels before it can be replenished. There is an interesting test, known as the Bryce-Smith zinc taste test (ZTT) [139], that is sometimes useful to gauge body zinc sufficiency, and here is how it works. You place about half a teaspoon of zinc sulphate solution in your mouth and swish it around for about 10 seconds. The objective is to experience a bitter taste somewhat immediately, indicating sufficient zinc, which is associated with the sense of taste. Delayed or no taste response is indicative of concomitantly lower zinc levels. Zinc sulphate solutions for use in this test are available from Biotics Research as Aqueous Zinc [94]. In the event of a deficiency, I have used zinc citrate and OptiZinc supplements (widely available).

The objective is to begin zinc supplementation and, about once per week, redo the taste test until the desired result is achieved; then reduce the supplementation to a maintenance dose. My personal experience has been that until magnesium levels are restored, it is impossible to pass this test, regardless of how much zinc is taken. I take 50 to 75 mg per day. Potassium supplementation is also usually required when magnesium levels have been depleted. My preference is to use potassium citrate (widely available), since it is also alkalizing. Note that anyone with impaired kidney function or who is taking diuretics should consult their doctor before using potassium supplements. If more than 1000 mg is required to maintain alkalinity during detoxing, blood testing of potassium levels is suggested.

I am not a fan of putting products on the skin that contain unnatural ingredients. However, there are some products with a low potential toxicity that can be used for a short period of time as an aid to restoring essential minerals and, for those, I make an exception. In the case of zinc, there are topical supplementation products available such as a zinc sulphate cream by Kirkman Labs [140].

While it would be great if we could normalize mineral levels just by taking supplements, this may not be possible because of the effect of toxins in our bodies. For example, mercury and other heavy metals along with Candida overgrowth can so derange mineral transport in the body that it is difficult to normalize magnesium, potassium, zinc and other essential minerals until the toxin load has been somewhat reduced. Therefore, the idea is to begin mineral repletion in parallel with detoxification (see *The Wellness Project* or *Nature's Detox Plan*).

Salt

I already discussed the availability of large quantities of salt from animal blood. Drinking blood is not convenient for me, so I supplement my diet with an unrefined ancient seabed salt. I avoid all refined salts such as common table salt and most other salts, even those labeled as "sea salt." In the unrefined category, there are those salts that are harvested from the ocean, and those that are harvested from ancient seabeds that have been buried for millions of years. The latter are my preference simply because of the currently contaminated state of our oceans, and the fact that we have yet to identify all of these contaminants, let alone measure them. In theory, ancient seabeds have been protected from modern pollution, and the odds are higher that they have avoided modern contaminants. The one I use is *RealSalt* from Redmond Incorporated in Utah [141]. There are some ancient seabed salts advertised from various other parts of the world, but I am skeptical of the quality control and test methods used.

Salt has the ability to cause the removal of toxins from the body in ways that we do not understand. I love salt, use it to taste, and estimate I consume about 2 grams per day. Am I worried about high blood pressure? No. My resting blood pressure ranges from 90/50 to 110/60. As far as I am concerned, none of the research relating salt intake to high blood pressure is applicable to the Original Diet, where we use only unrefined salt, and eliminate all of the toxic foods. There simply are no studies for those conditions, except of course for the 99,000-generation one. An excellent book on the healthy aspects of salt, also showing that, for the most part, the increase in blood pressure from salt is a transient one, is *Salt: Your Way to Health* by David Brownstein [142].

Glandulars

While we have already discussed liver, not a lot of folks like to eat the other organs of animals. Adrenals, thyroid, lung, and spleen, to mention a few, just do not sound appetizing. Therefore, unlike PA, we are thus missing some fatty acids, beneficial hormones, enzymes, and probably a whole lot more. We know there are benefits to be obtained because natural thyroid hormones from cow or pig are widely prescribed to people with low functioning thyroid glands.

To partially make up for my lack of raw organ/gland intake, I take a multi-glandular supplement, which is a freeze-dried version of the various glands from clean, naturally fed animals. There is scant evidence as to what survives processing in these products, but it is one way to hedge bets in this area. One I have used is Neonatal Multi-Gland by Biotics Research [94], containing spleen, heart, pancreas, kidney, brain, liver, adrenal, thymus, intestine, eye, and pituitary. I take two per meal.

An interesting event happened in my house that buttressed my appreciation of glandulars. I previously mentioned our cats, raised on a raw food diet that includes as many glands and other organs as we can obtain, along with a glandular supplement. However, it is not a perfect rat. One day when I was in the kitchen preparing lunch I had put my supplements, including two glandular tablets, on the table and turned my attention to the oven for a couple of minutes. When I returned, all the vitamins were on the floor, but upon retrieving them, I noticed that only the glandulars were missing. It finally occurred to me that the cats, who were hanging around, had eaten them. As an experiment, I ground up a tablet and put it in front of the two cats. Whoosh - gone in a second! I repeated the experiment using the desiccated liver discussed above, with the same result. Usually, the cats are quite leisurely when they eat, but they gobbled up the glandulars, leading to the conclusion that they needed more than what was in their diet, so we have upped the amount.

As a result of toxins in the body, both adrenal and thyroid gland malfunction has become widespread, and a plethora of supplements are available, each claiming to support the gland in some manner. With respect to thyroid glandulars, the ones sold without prescription are required to have the hormone thyroxine (T4) removed. For a non-prescription natural thyroid extract, I have used GTA-Forte II from Biotics Research [94]. In the prescription category, there are synthetics and natural, usually extracts from pig glands. In keeping with the Original Diet, for thyroid hormone supplementation to treat a hypothyroid condition, the natural form would be preferable. The popular prescription natural brands are Armour® and Westhroid®, and there are several good websites describing the differences [143] [144]. There is a lot more discussion about the thyroid in the iodine and halogen portions of *The Wellness Project*. With respect to adrenal glandulars, for a non-prescription natural whole adrenal extract, I have used Cytozyme-AD from Biotics Research. It is a source of neonatal bovine whole adrenal gland.

Gelatin

Gelatin is found in the skin and bones of animals, including mammals, fowl, and fish, and broth made from animal bones is a good source of gelatin. Contrary to popular belief, hoofs, horns, hair, feathers, or any keratin material is not a source of gelatin. For those not inclined to consume bone soup, a gelatin supplement is suggested. Most of us are familiar with gelatin in the form of desserts such as Jell-O®, but gelatin has many health benefits that make it an important part of the Original Diet. Gelatin is related to collagen, which may be thought of as the glue that hold our body together and is critical to bone, joint and skin health. The amino acids glycine and proline, found in abundance in gelatin, play an important role in building cartilage and preventing bone disorders [145]. Glycine is one of the amino acids necessary to form glutathione, an important peptide used to remove a variety of toxins from the body. Glycine also helps digestion by enhancing gastric acid secretion [146], an important factor in the protein digestion process, as discussed more fully in the digestive rehabilitation section below.

Gelatin, which mostly consists of protein, was given a bad name several years ago when it was discovered that it could not be used as a complete meal replacement because it was not a complete protein and was missing or weak in a few amino acids. Of course, gelatin was never meant to be eaten alone in the context of PA's diet. It was again given a bad name during the mad-cow scare, when it was thought that commercial gelatin could be contaminated. Many studies were conducted to show that gelatin rendered from animal skin and bones was not at risk, and the processing steps used to make gelatin further reduce any potential risks [147]. The majority of supplement capsules are made from gelatin.

The definitive references on the nutritional benefits of gelatin come from articles by Dr. Francis Pottenger, mentioned earlier in connection with his raw cat food studies, and the book *Gelatin in*

Nutrition and Medicine by N. R. Gotthoffer [96], which includes much of the gelatin research conducted in the 19th century. The following are some of Gotthoffer's findings, which have also been reported by Kaayla Daniel in the article *Why Broth is Beautiful*, published in Wise Traditions by the Weston A. Price Foundation, Spring 2003, Volume 4, No. 1 [7].

Early in the 20th century, researchers showed that gelatin increases the utilization of the protein in wheat, oats, and barley, though not of corn; that the digestibility of beans is vastly improved with the addition of gelatin; and that gelatin helps the digestion of meat protein. The last appears to confirm the subjective reports of many people who say that meats found in soups and pot roasts--cooked with bones for a long time in a liquid to which a touch of vinegar has been added--are easier to digest than quickly cooked steaks and chops, and why gelatin-rich gravies are at the heart of many culinary traditions.

Gotthoffer reports the existence of more than 30 years of research studies showing that gelatin can improve the digestion of milk and milk products. Accordingly, nutrition textbook writers of the 1920s and 1930s recommended that gelatin be included in infant formulas to help bring cow's milk closer to human milk. Apparently, gelatin exerted a very important influence on the milk fat. It served not only to emulsify the fat but also, by stabilizing the casein, improved the digestibility and absorption of the fat, which otherwise would be carried down with casein in a lumpy mass. As a result, infants fed gelatin-enriched formulas showed reduced allergic symptoms, vomiting, colic, diarrhea, constipation, and respiratory ailments than those on straight cow's milk.

Gelatin's reputation as a health restorer includes its ability to soothe the GI tract and to dramatically improve rheumatoid arthritis as well as other degenerative joint conditions and inflammatory bowel diseases [148]. It has also been reported that gelatin will protect gastric mucosal integrity, at least in lab rats subjected to ethanol-induced mucosal damage [149]. Another study showed that collagen hydrolysate, an extract of gelatin, reduced pain in patients with osteoarthritis of the knee or hip and that gelatin held a significant treatment advantage over the placebo [150].

As you can see from the above, I think very highly of gelatin, which has been largely ignored by the mainstream medical community in favor of drugs. As a supplement, used in place of bone broth, I use Beef

Gelatin made by Great Lakes Gelatin Company [151]. Gelatin is a tasteless and odorless powder that mixes well in hot water. One teaspoon (about 5 grams) per meal is a suitable starting dose.

Essential Fatty Acids

According to the medical community, the essential fatty acids (EFAs) for humans are certain polyunsaturated fatty acids (PUFAs) in the omega-6 and omega-3 families, and they must be obtained from the diet. The body needs them for many foundational purposes, such as building healthy cell membranes, a properly functioning brain, and for a whole gamut of hormone-like substances that regulate, among other things, immune and inflammatory responses.

The alternative health community has bombarded us with a message stating the "importance" of getting enough omega-3 fatty acids in our (SAD) diet, by using supplements such as fish oils and flax seed oil. In the following discussion, you will see why omega-3 supplements are not only not required on the Original Diet, they should be avoided because they can promote illness by generating substantial amounts of toxins.

Let's see what these oils are supposed to nutritionally accomplish. There seems to be general agreement that the SAD diet has a preponderance of omega-6 fatty acids in it, as compared to omega-3s. Many studies, including some Paleo diet studies indicate that a healthy range of omega-6 to omega-3 is from about 1:1 to 4:1, but the SAD diet ratios are usually way over 10:1. A classic study of rats showed that the optimum ratio to maintain learning skills and resistance to pain was 4:1 [152]. The omega-6 overload in the SAD diet comes mostly from nut and seed oils, products consumed in great quantity in the modern diet, but are non-existent in the Original Diet, as is this whole issue of having to balance the two fatty acid groups. Many illnesses are being ascribed to this modern ratio imbalance, and we are told to increase dramatically our omega-3 intake to compensate for the omega-6 excess. As an astute reader, you may well ask why one would not just reduce the omega-6 dietary intake to solve the ratio problem, but to do that would gut the SAD diet of much of its devotees' favorite foods, and, gosh, it would start to look like the Original Diet.

On the Original Diet, including Tier One and Two food choices, PA would have obtained the EFAs primarily from animal sources. The omega-3s would have been obtained from grass-fed muscle meat and in larger amounts from eating the brains, liver and other organs of prey. It is my contention that the Original Diet provides all of the EFAs the body needs, and in the proper ratio. No EFA supplements are needed, and it may be detrimental to add any of them. I could (and should) stop right here and not waste any more time on this issue, but it has been so highly hyped in the media that I feel compelled to put in my two-cents worth. What follows is a summary of my research into the omega-3 supplement industry, followed by a discussion of how the Original Diet avoids all of the pitfalls I encountered.

I have found it very frustrating in dealing with the oil supplement industry – they seem to win the prize when it comes to hiding the ball. Let's start at the beginning. There is general agreement that the essential fatty acids, particularly the omega-3s, are indeed fragile, and most oil products that contain them, such as the seed-based oils like flax seed and its blends, and the fish and fish liver (usually cod liver) oils, caution the consumer to "refrigerate after opening," to consume the refrigerated oil in a few weeks, and to not use it for cooking. By fragile I mean they easily become oxidized or rancid. Some brands boast of having the container back-filled with nitrogen to prevent oxidative damage from air. Still others boast of being in a dark container (opaque plastic or brown glass) to protect against light damage. The message to the consumer is loud and clear – these oils are easily damaged by exposure to heat, light and air. If only the manufacturers would heed their own advice. Flax seed and fish oils in their natural state have high omega-3 content, and virtually no omega-6 content. Starting with flax (linseed) seeds, let's look at the processing of the oil. There are various ways to get the oil out of the seed, including the use of chemical solvents such as hexane, and the use of mechanical presses to squeeze the oil out.

While solvents are still used for many vegetable oils, they are in disfavor in the health arena because they tend to combine with seed and oil compounds to produce toxic stuff, and sometimes require evaporation temperatures way above that of boiling water, not a smart thing to do with heat-sensitive oils. Expeller pressing, sometimes called "cold pressing" is now the preferred method. There is no definition in the U.S. for cold pressing, and in some cases "cold" is actually quite hot, above the temperature of boiling water. Some oils are further refined, such as by being bleached, and deodorized. Flaxseeds are not digestible in the shell (as Nature intended), but you could get the omega-3s directly from the flax seeds by grinding them yourself and eating the pulp. Unfortunately, the grinding operation might well heat the seeds significantly, so then you would be eating rancid seed pulp. In any case, you would be eating the natural toxins MA put in there to keep you from eating her seeds.

As you can see, seed oil processing is fraught with potential problems in which the oil may be subjected to the high temperatures consumers are cautioned against, and for good reason. The scientific community is still discovering the many ways in which heating and otherwise processing oils makes them toxic to humans. It started with hydrogenation, a true Frankenmethod of hardening vegetables oils, which led to the creation of trans-fats, which are now the bad fats du jour.

The lipid industry has made some valiant attempts to quantify the purity of food oils. As an example, efforts have been made to quantify the oxidation of fats and oils (the rancidity) by defining the Peroxide Index (PV). Well, they found this was not accurate enough to detect all forms of rancidity, so they added the Anisidine Value (AV), which alone is also not sufficient. Then they defined the Totox Value (TV), which is AV + 2PV. I am not a lipid chemist, but this numbers game makes me nervous. They have yet to make a dent in defining, measuring, or determining the other types of damage resulting from the processing of polyunsaturated oils and their effect on the human body, such as cyclic fatty acid derivatives, cross-linked fatty acid chains, dimers, polymers, cross-linked triglycerides, body-shifted molecules, and molecular fragments. The bottom line for me with respect to seed oils is this: in keeping with the precepts of the Original Diet, I do not want to mess with MA's seeds, and I do not need to on the Original Diet. A caveat is also in order here. For those on the Original Diet, which does not have an omega-6 overload, taking large amounts of a seed or seed oil like flax seed can be counterproductive, as it contains a lot of omega-3 but almost no omega-6, thus upsetting the diet ratio in the reverse direction (too much omega-3). See the book *Fats That Heal and Fats That Kill* by Udo Erasmus for a discussion of the dangers of this imbalance [153].

Onward to the fish-oil industry. Here we have plain fish oils extracted from the flesh, and liver oils extracted from the liver. Many of the same steps used in vegetable oil processing are also used here, including solvents and pressing. However, fish oils face an additional hurdle. As discussed above, virtually all fish are contaminated with heavy metals such as mercury and arsenic, as well as pesticides and organic contaminants such as PCBs. I have been told by industry representatives that the flesh contains most of the heavy metals, and the liver contains most of the pesticides and organic contaminants. Either way, there are basically two choices presented to the consumer: molecular distillation, a high temperature process used to remove contaminants; or un-distilled oil, which still contains the contaminants. In the flesh-derived fish oil business, the distillation process predominates, but the effect of heating the oil to high temperatures required for distillation may well result in damaged fatty acids, detrimental to health, and possibly leaving the consumer with clean but heat-damaged oil that, after the fact, one is now told to keep in the refrigerator!

There are non-distilled oils such as salmon oil that still contain contaminants, so that is the risk factor in this category. Other than various regulatory agencies such as WHO (World Health Organization) and the EPA (Environmental Protection Agency) and the FDA and the USDA (U. S. Department of Agriculture) putting some numbers down on paper, we are clueless as to safe contaminant limits. The agencies, some supported by the fishing industry, are still bickering as to whose numbers are right. Another of these non-distilled oils is made from krill, small plankton that is reputed to have low levels of contaminants, and claims are made that high heat is not used for extraction. From what I could find in my research, the krill oil extraction process that appears to be used for some brands is that disclosed in U.S. Patent 6,800,299, involving a solvent-based system using ketones, which is probably an improvement over hexane. However, as stated in the literature, the issue with using solvent extraction is not only the solvent itself, but toxic compounds that can be formed between the solvent and the compounds in the oil [31].

Moving along to fish liver oil, in its natural form it could be ingested as a source of omega-3s in place of eating animal brain or liver. It has the advantage of not only containing the usual omega-3 fatty acids, but also the long chain varieties, such as DHA (Docosahexaenoic Acid), found in human and animal brains and to a lesser extent in their livers. Another nice feature of unprocessed fish liver is that it contains natural versions of vitamins A and D in a well-balanced ratio. Here again, as a supplement, the oil choices are molecularly distilled or un-distilled. Virtually all are distilled, which has the unfortunate effect of destroying most of the natural vitamins A and D, so these nutrients are added back in synthetic form, and in ratios that suit the whims of the manufacturer. At least one producer claims to remove the natural vitamins before distillation, and then return them afterward, using a proprietary process. The only process I could find for extracting vitamins from oil is to use solvents. Lastly, there is a recent market addition to the liver oil selection that uses fermentation to produce un-distilled oil, but the contaminant problem remains. An excellent article on the cod liver oil processing industry can be found on the Weston Price Foundation website [7].

I am not comfortable with any fish oil supplements currently on the market, and personally avoid them for the following reasons: while there is not a wealth of information on the subject, I feel quite strongly that putting damaged fatty acids into one's body is a very bad thing to do, particularly because of its impact on the cardiovascular system. Oxidized fatty acids are known to predispose one toward arterial plaque, and I doubt they have a favorable effect on the brain, which is mostly fat. I also do not have sufficient confidence in the lipid chemists that they know how to detect, measure, and evaluate the health consequences of damaged fats. It took them decades to figure out (or admit to) the problems inherent with hydrogenation and trans-fats. I also am not a fan of consuming environmentally contaminated fish products, and government agency "safe" levels on a piece of paper (frequently revised) also give me no comfort. Finally, the fact that the vitamins A and D in virtually all fish liver oils are actually the same synthetic stuff you can buy in a supplement bottle contributes to my lack of enthusiasm for commercially available fish oils.

Yet, there are many, many cases where people taking omega-3 supplements feel better. To see how it is possible that these oils are *healthy* (a comparative term) even if they may be damaged, we need to consider the latest thoughts on how the body processes damaged fats. The supposition is that when a person ingests a damaged fatty acid, say a trans-fat-damaged version of an omega-6 fat, the body will put it in a site reserved for undamaged omega-6 fats, either because it cannot tell the difference, or because a damaged omega-6 is better than none at all. This characteristic can go one step further to translocation – if one does not take in enough omega-3 fats to satisfy the body's needs and instead takes in too many omega-6s, the body can start putting the omega-6s into the omega-3 sites.

So, now let's take the typical case of a person on the SAD diet, overloaded with omega-6s, most of which are damaged due to typical food processing (such as frying with unsaturated vegetable oils). We can presume the body has loaded all of the omega-6 and probably most of the omega-3 receptor sites with the ingested damaged omega-6s. Along comes some damaged omega-3 fish oil, and this person starts to take some. Well, the body can now put these damaged omega-3s into omega-3 sites in place of damaged omega-6s – quite an improvement, so the person feels better, and even the mostly meaningless blood tests show improvement. Voila, they are getting *healthy* (actually, less unhealthy). This is another example of how removing the bad stuff can make you somewhat less unhealthy as compared to your present state of health, even if you are replacing it with less than good stuff. This may be good enough for some people, in which case I encourage them to continue down this path.

The goal of The Original Diet, however, is to put in the good stuff and leave out the bad stuff. Sure, the body can process some amount of damaged fats eaten each day and get rid of them, but that takes defense system energy better reserved for more serious tasks such as eliminating cancer cells and fending off unwanted bacteria, viruses and yeasts. Why deliberately put in bad stuff if you don't have to? With this in mind, let's now take a look at the Original Diet and the need, if any, for essential fatty acid supplementation.

It would be nice to know the daily requirement for the essential fatty acids, but all of the efforts to estimate those are based on people who eat the SAD diet, and are thus not useful for our purpose. A major reason, discussed earlier, is that the large intake of damaged omega-6 from the SAD diet necessitates large offsetting amounts of omega-3. However, we can get some meaningful data from EFA studies of infant diets, where the total intake of fatty acids can be closely controlled. An EFA amount of as little as 0.1% of total calories appeared to be sufficient to prevent a variety of symptoms associated with EFA deficiency [154]. On a 2000-calorie daily food intake, this translates to a total of about 225 mg of EFAs. For purposes of discussion, let's use a 4:1 ratio and assign 225 mg to the omega-6 intake and 55 mg to the omega-3 intake as safe daily dietary levels to avoid deficiency.

In the Original Diet, research shows we obtain substantial amounts of omega-3 and -6 fatty acids in a proper ratio from our grass-fed meat [155]. If we ate clean liver, such as broiled calf's liver (not fried), this would be an added boost to both the -3 and -6 category, including the long chains. I understand the "Mad Cow" threat is a strong deterrent, but animal brain would yield even more omega-3s. Actually, in the Original Diet, grass-fed muscle meat alone produces ideal fatty acid ratios and more omega-3s than fish flesh. Beef and lamb liver are also excellent sources of omega-3s. A 1998 study of the fatty acid composition of grass fed beef and lamb liver found that 100 grams (about 3 ounces) contained 151 milligrams of EPA and 83 milligrams of DHA, and an omega6/3 ratio of 0.71[75]. For those who are not liver lovers, I already discussed a freeze-dried liver supplement that contains the fatty acids, and it may be a suitable EFA (Essential Fatty Acid) supplement.

If one wants to up the amount of essential fatty acids in the Original Diet, including the long-chain ones, a suggestion is already on the Original Diet list of supplementary foods: EGGS. In particular, I am referring to eggs from free-range hens fed a variety of natural foods that enhance their fatty acid profile in the right direction, producing healthy omega-6 to -3 ratios, and also yielding substantial DHA and EPA long-chain fatty acids. A suggested brand is labeled Christopher Eggs, and they are available at a wide range of markets [156]. I would avoid eating conventional grain-fed penned-hen eggs. Their fatty acid omega-6/omega-3 profile is close to 20:1, much like grain-fed beef. An interesting analogy can be made here. Remember the discussion above about how ruminants such as cows process toxic or indigestible plant matter like grass (their natural food), into something nontoxic that we are able to assimilate, like meat? Well, here we have chickens, whose natural food sources include seeds such as flax seed, which they are genetically designed to process, providing us with a food we can assimilate – eggs.

Studies have been conducted on the fatty acid profile of egg yolks from chickens fed a high omega-3 seed diet, like flax seeds, and the results show omega-6/omega-3 ratios around 3:1, as well as high levels of DHA [157]. In fact, a single one of these egg yolks can provide more than enough EFAs to meet the daily requirement on the Original Diet. I avoid omega-3 supplements such as fish and flax oils while on the Original Diet in order not to disturb the fatty acid ratio of the diet in the wrong direction of excess omega-3, leading to some very nasty symptoms.

From the above discussion, it is apparent that no EFA supplements are needed with the Original Diet. Further, there is evidence that increasing the PUFA intake above the small amounts necessary can be very detrimental one's health. As previously mentioned, PUFAs are very easily oxidized, and once oxidized in the body, they promote oxidative stress as a result of lipid peroxidation, which is another way of saying that they produce toxic substances in the body that significantly burden its defense system. It appears that the body will attempt to convert excess PUFAs into saturated fat, but inevitably dietary PUFAs still accumulate over time in cells and can increase the risk of cancer [158]. A multi-institutional prospective study in 2004 concluded that heart disease was directly correlated with PUFA intake, and inversely correlated with intake of saturated fat [159]. This study is sometimes referred to as the "American Paradox" because there are many other studies that appear to show the contrary. Antioxidants such as the vitamin E complex can sometimes slow the oxidative damage. Because of the inconsistent data on the effects of excessive PUFA intake, it would seem to make sense to minimize such intake. However, the thrust of the alternative health campaign is just devoted to balancing fatty acid ratios - add more omega-3 supplements to offset high omega-6 intake - while ignoring the absolute amounts of each being ingested. This may well backfire in the future if it eventually becomes apparent that the total amount of PUFAs consumed is as important as, or perhaps more important than the ratio, when it comes to the overall health of the person. Which brings me to a discussion of sesame seeds.

Researchers have found that eating sesame seeds can shut down the body's ability to make a crucial fatty acid that makes up about 50 % of our brain. A lignan (a phytoestrogen) called sesamin in sesame seeds interferes with an enzyme, delta 5 desaturase, which is part of the pathway that makes arachidonic acid (AA) from dietary intake of omega-6 linoleic acid. If that pathway is disrupted, there is a potential of shutting down at least a portion of AA production (the brain is about 50% AA). Doing so also upsets the amount of DHA that the body makes from omega-3 linolenic acid using that same enzyme, potentially increasing DHA production. The supplement community thinks this is great and actually puts sesamin in supplements for this very reason. You see, on the SAD diet, one gets too much AA and not enough DHA, so this is their way to fix it. Another way, of course, is to stop eating all of the seeds in the first place, since they are a major dietary cause of the problem, but that does not result in profits. Well, I can tell you that it could be bad news to eat sesame seeds on the Original Diet, which already has a natural fatty acid balance, because it could easily cause an AA deficiency [160] [161]. The point of this little excursion was to indicate how easily some of the foods in a SAD diet, like seeds, can mess with our fatty acid balance in unpredictable ways.

Speculating beyond sesame seeds, I wonder if some other plant food, (or maybe even sesame seeds) that we excluded from the Original Diet as naturally toxic, might result in *saturated* fat causing some detrimental effect on health in the SAD diet. Let us say, hypothetically, that we accept as correct the studies showing that people that eat a SAD diet and have high intake of saturated fat have a higher risk of heart disease. First, that is very different than saying saturated fat causes heart disease. What may have been proven in these studies, if anything, is that if you eat a lot of saturated fat while also eating seeds, vegetables, dairy, processed oils, sugars, artificial sweeteners and tap water, it is unhealthy. I have already speculated above on the saturated fat/magnesium deficiency connection, and magnesium deficiency is rampant among SAD eaters. Those heart disease studies on saturated fats are not relevant to the Original Diet, where all of the toxic foods (like sesame seeds) have been eliminated, and magnesium is provided in adequate amounts.

It would be interesting to conduct studies to see which of the SAD diet components, if any, is the culprit in messing with saturated fat, just as they found that sesame seeds messed with polyunsaturated fats. My guess would be that it is also a seed-related compound, because the SAD diet is filled with foods from seeds. All grains are seeds (bread, pasta, cake, cookies, pizza, rice, etc.), and many are cooked using seed oils (canola, safflower, peanut). Well, if you eat MA's seeds (the reproductive agents of plants) in great quantity, this might be another way that it makes you sick so that you will cut it out.

My speculation regarding saturated fat and magnesium deficiency fits perfectly in the above model involving seeds. It works like this: seeds contain natural toxins that bind up minerals in the body, including magnesium, contributing to magnesium depletion. Saturated fat also binds with magnesium, aggravating depletion, which is a major culprit in heart disease. This is a fertile area for research, but it would have to be privately funded since it does not lead to the sale of any products other than magnesium supplements.

Chapter 12 - Digestive Rehabilitation

This section is for people intrigued with the Original Diet, but who have had digestive problems in the past eating meat. The best way to make the transition from a SAD diet to the Original Diet is to do so slowly, introducing small amounts of easily digested meat, such as ground patties into the diet, while also starting to drop some of the SAD foods. This process can take many months, but is the most natural way to go. Remember that during the transition, a huge toxic load is being removed from the body in the form of MA's naturally occurring toxins. The body can actually go through a "die-off reaction." The upshot of this is that one can feel lousy during the transition as the body adjusts to its natural diet. Further, some established parasitic toxins in the body, particularly Candida, get very unhappy when deprived of their favorite foods (which you will be giving up), and this can make one feel quite miserable until they are dealt with.

Many folks who have been, or are dealing with Candida overgrowth know that grains, sugars, and alcohol are the troubling foods. Having dealt with Candida issues for most of my life, I spend a great deal of time discussing it in *The Wellness Project*. Fruit is sometimes identified as a problem Candida food. On the Original Diet, eating only limited amounts of carbs (typically less than 75 grams per day) in the form of whole fresh fruit (no dried fruit and no fruit juice), and taking the spore-forming bacteria seems to work quite well when combined with suitable fungal detoxification programs.

Having said that, there are people who exhibit allergic reactions to certain fruit, including those that pass the ABC test. Examples are watermelon, figs, cherimoya and mango. Symptoms include itching, rashes, nasal congestion, and asthma-like reactions. Researchers have coined the term "latex-fruit syndrome" in an effort to explain this phenomenon [162]. They have found that many of those who exhibit this syndrome also have an allergic reaction to natural rubber latex, usually first detected upon exposure to latex gloves. Interestingly, several of the proteins believed responsible for the allergic reactions possess potent antifungal characteristics. Examples of such proteins are chitinases and glucanases, both capable of rupturing yeast cells.

Yeast overgrowth in the body, particularly Candida, is a major obstacle to health, and rupture of those cells can produce all of the symptoms listed above for the latex-fruit syndrome. Personally, when I (unknowingly) had such a yeast overgrowth many years ago, I was allergic to certain fruits such as peaches and watermelon, and I used to get canker sores from eating citrus fruit. Now that the yeast is under control, all of those symptoms have disappeared, highlighting the importance of detoxification and its interaction with diet. Incidentally, all of my pollen allergies also disappeared, such as ragweed allergy and hay fever. So for those with fruit allergies, until you can implement some of the detox protocols of *The Wellness Project*, avoid or minimize eating those fruits known to produce symptoms. There is also some evidence that peeling the fruit, such as apples and peaches, before eating, can reduce or eliminate symptoms [163].

Beef allergy is considered to be very rare (pun intended), and I wonder how many of the few cases may be reacting to growth hormones or other adulterations found in conventional meat. I would venture that eating organic grass-fed free-range meat, along with detoxification, would eliminate even the few cases of meat allergy. As already mentioned, later introduced animal products such as chicken do have a record of allergy prevalence.

Some other roadblocks in the way of a smooth diet transition are a lack of hydrochloric (HCl) acid, a digestive secretion produced in the stomach; lack of digestive enzymes, mostly produced in the pancreas, and lack of bile, produced in the liver and stored in the gall bladder. Some of these shortages can be caused by many years on a SAD diet which did not required digestive support from these organs, and hence they have fallen into disuse (use it or lose it). In other instances, this digestive difficulty may be caused by various infections, such as H.pylori (Helicobacter Pylori) and Candida overgrowth, either of which could also be due to eating the SAD diet. Then there are all of the environmental and medical/dental-induced contaminants such as heavy metals and organic poisons that can wreak havoc with digestion. Those are discussed in *The Wellness Project*. There is also some evidence that blood type has an influence, with type A generally having lower stomach acid levels than type O.

For individuals interested in making the diet switch, some digestive supplements might help pave the way during the transition, although I suggest that you use them only for a limited time. A caveat, however, is in order. Depending on the ultimate causes of digestive disturbances, these supplements may work fine, may not work at all, or may make digestive symptoms worse, possibly as a result of toxins in the body. In other words, you should always be mindful of how your body is reacting to any type of supplementation and proceed conservatively.

Bitters/Betaine HCL/Digestive Enzymes

Herbal bitters have been used for years as a remedy for digestive ailments, so let's look at these first. We know all about bitters from MA because of our fruit discussion, and we know we have separate taste buds just for bitter taste. Most digestive bitters are liquid preparations of the very parts of the plants that are avoided on the Original Diet because they are very likely to be toxic. From my point of view, this is why bitters seem to work to "wake up" the digestive system. This is a guess, of course, but consider that when the bitters are placed on our tongue and hit our bitter-taste buds, our bodies are programmed to expect that a load of toxic plant material is about to hit our stomach. In defense, the body starts cranking acid, pepsin, digestive enzymes and anything else it can throw at the stuff to try to detoxify it. On the one hand, this is a clever way to reawaken the digestive system using a natural process. On the other hand, we may be stressing the body unnecessarily to go on alert. Yet another concern is whether we are behavior conditioning our digestive system to awaken only when we consume something bitter. As a short-term solution, say only for a few months, perhaps this method could be used, for example, during the diet switchover period. There are many herbal bitter concoctions on the market for digestive relief, some of which are labeled Swedish bitters, and they are quite popular in Europe.

Instead of bitters, another approach is to approximate nature by directly replacing the missing elements in our digestive system. Let's start with HCl, which, when not sufficiently available, causes digestive upset and heartburn. Yet if you tell your doctor you have heartburn, he/she will probably give you an acid-suppressing drug or recommend antacids, which are a big business. Research, however, tells us that antacids don't really benefit you in the long run, and can lead to helicobacter pylori overgrowth (the cause of ulcers), pneumonia, and tuberculosis, just for starters. For a good discussion of the need for stomach acid see the book : *Why Stomach Acid Is Good For You* by Jonathan Wright [164].

Insufficient HCl is commonly blamed on aging and in some cases blood type (those with blood type A seems to have lower amounts than blood type O), but it could also be a result of accumulated toxins in the system, including those resulting from a poor diet. A supplement used for insufficient HCl is betaine HCl, a product widely available in health food stores, and it usually includes pepsin, a digestive enzyme also produced in the stomach. It should be taken with a meal, and the dosage is determined experimentally, varying from about 130 mg to several grams per meal. The goal is to simulate nature's wonderful system of secreting just the right amount for each meal, which varies with the meal size and content. At best, this is going to end up as a crude approximation, but fortunately, we are not after perfection. Anyone with a stomach ulcer should avoid this supplement until the ulcer is healed. One brand of Betaine HCL caps (with pepsin) is Twinlab [165].

There are a few tests available to determine stomach pH, and thus, indirectly, the need for HCl supplementation, but each has its drawbacks, so one can just start taking some small amounts of Betaine HCl and see what effect it has on digestion. If a warm sensation in the gut is experienced while eating after taking the supplement, this may indicate an excessive amount of HCl, so the dose is reduced until the sensation is eliminated. A burning sensation is a sign to stop taking it temporarily, and instead take some supplements that may be helpful to heal an inflamed stomach, such as slippery elm, discussed below.

An HCl supplement with pepsin helps the body break down protein, among other things and, in theory, you will be able to tolerate animal products without discomfort, even if they haven't been eaten for a long period of time. This supplement can also help resolve a vicious digestive cycle. Here's the picture: with insufficient stomach acid, one cannot assimilate all of their food efficiently and, thus, they may not absorb certain nutritional elements, particularly minerals such as zinc, necessary for the production of stomach acid in the first place. For instance, the body needs chloride, which is from salt, and zinc and other minerals often deficient in today's refined diets. The HCl supplement jumpstarts the digestive processes and when the body's own levels come up, the digestive system should be able to resume the acid production operation on its own. In the above discussion of gelatin, it was mentioned that it could be used to correct stomach acid deficiencies. As an integral component of the Original Diet, I view gelatin as an important ingredient for the correction of HCl deficiency in the long-term.

A special note is in order here regarding dolomite, which contains minerals in their carbonate form, requiring HCl or some other acid for assimilation. As explained above, taking dolomite with magnesium taurate away from meals helps with acid production. If you know you are deficient in stomach acid, take the dolomite with one tablet of *HCL-Plus* by Biotics Research [94]. It supplies a small amount of HCl, insuring full assimilation.

Another way to improve digestion is with a digestive enzyme supplement. The body naturally produces digestive enzymes to break down food. Some are produced in the mouth while chewing food, and others are made in the gut and in the pancreas as food enters the stomach and small intestine. These enzymes have different roles. Some help to break down protein, still others break down fats, and others carbohydrates. Those who have followed a primarily vegetarian diet may be short on the enzymes that digest protein (proteases) and fat (lipases), and a deficiency can lead to indigestion, discomfort, and an inability to assimilate all of the food. People tend not to be deficient in the carbohydrate enzymes (amylases).

There is some controversy about whether enzyme supplements become habit-forming and prevent the body from gearing up its own. I haven't seen that happen, but I would only take them during the diet transition period. Further, some fruits in the Original Diet contain digestive enzymes, making it even less likely that the body will shut down its own ability to make enzymes from ingesting them in supplement form. In the animal world, the pancreas of an animal would be a source of digestive enzymes if, in fact, PA consumed the pancreas. From my point of view, it is much more likely that PA's supplementary digestive enzymes came from fruit. Tropical fruits such as papaya (papain) and pineapple (bromelain) are typically the source for plant-based protease enzyme supplements. Well, wouldn't you know it, these fruit enzyme profiles fit perfectly into the Original Diet.

For an enzyme supplement during the diet transition phase, I would eat papaya (but only if it is labeled as not genetically modified) and/or pineapple with meals, to help digest meat protein. A second choice is to get papain or bromelain in the form of supplements and take those with meals– there are many brands. Look for those where the only ingredient is papaya or pineapple. Usually, portions of the fruit that are not on the Original Diet are used, such as the leaf or a part of the unripe fruit. Since this supplement is for short-term use, I don't have a problem with this implementation. Because of the GMO issues with papaya, I prefer a bromelain supplement. One example is Bromelain by Now Foods, available in tablet or capsule form, and one per meal is a good starting dose [112]. If the enzymes work, one should experience better bowel movements as well as less bloat and discomfort after eating. For those with an inflamed gut, however, protein-digesting enzymes can aggravate the condition, requiring one to stop or severely cut back on dosage if gut pain or headaches are experienced. In such case, see the section below regarding gut repair.

It is interesting to note that there are two distinct ways in which digestive enzymes can be used. One is to help digest food, in which case, the enzymes are taken with food. The second usage is aimed at digesting certain proteins present in the bloodstream, some of which may have originated as remnants of undigested food, and which are involved in inflammation and allergic reactions. Some people target these proteins in an effort to help reduce inflammation, pain, and allergies, simply by taking the enzyme supplements between meals. The goal, of course, is only to use the supplements during your transition to the Original Diet. After a time, the combination of eating the right types of fruits and one's own pancreas waking up should make you digestively self-reliant.

Bile salts

Another digestive area that may need supplementing is the gall bladder, which could have either gone to sleep and/or been congested by being misused on the SAD diet. Unfortunately, many people have already had it removed because of gallstones and/or a strange notion within the medical community that people don't really need it, but they do. The liver makes bile, which is then stored and concentrated in the gall bladder between meals. The bile is then secreted into the small intestine to emulsify fats and get them into a form that the body can assimilate and utilize. This function is particularly important when eating animal fats. Some indications of insufficiency are pale stools, perhaps gray in color (bile gives our stool its characteristic brown color), and/or floating stools, which are full of undigested fat. Bile is an important pathway for the excretion of toxins, hence an insufficiency of bile can impair the ability to detoxify.

For those with a gall bladder, bile salt tablets may be useful as a supplement to ease the transition to animal fats. The protocol recommended by the supplement manufacturers is to cycle doses to avoid dependence upon the salts. They suggest starting with one tablet with meals the first day, two tablets with meals the second day, three on the third, and then back to one tablet the next day. Going up and down like this apparently prevents a dependence on the bile salts during the diet transition period, after which the gall bladder should be functioning normally. For those without a gall bladder, they suggest that one to two tablets with each meal is generally effective and can be used for life. Examples of bile salt supplements are Beta Plus by Biotics Research [94], and Cholacol by Standard Process [166]. Checking stool characteristics and tracking gastric symptoms would be a good way to monitor progress.

Probiotics

In the mucous lining of your intestinal tract is a teeming world of bacteria, fungi and other microorganisms. It is estimated that hundreds of species are present, some detrimental, some beneficial, and others than can become either, depending on the circumstances. These creatures number in the countless billions, more in fact, than the total number of cells in the body. If all of them were piled together, they would tip the scales at several pounds.

As of the writing of this book, we still have not identified the majority of the microbes in our gut, but a government-funded initiative has been officially announced that is planning to do just that. It is known as the NIH (National Institutes of Health) Human Microbiome Project, and their objectives include determining whether individuals share a core human microbiome, and trying to understand whether changes in the human microbiome can be correlated with changes in human health. Recently, there has been a renewed interest in gut microflora and its role in illness and inflammation [167], and I predict they will find it to be an important link in the riddles of illness.

The gut microorganisms that are carried around 24/7 in the body (but actually outside of it because the intestines from the mouth to the anus are actually outside the body, separated by the intestinal wall) are pivotal to quality of life and it's the balance among them that is vital to your existence in ways you never imagined. They can include bacteria, viruses, fungi, and a variety of parasites including worms, amoeba, and protozoa. In reality, all of these could be considered as parasites because many live off us, the host. Healthy bodies supposedly harbor huge colonies of so-called friendly bacteria, otherwise known as beneficial intestinal flora. The most famous of these bacterial "good guys" is the lactobacillus genus, among them the acidophilus strain, which is active in the lower portion of the small intestine. Bifidobacteria, another genus of bacteria, is primarily active in the colon. In addition are the spore-formers, which should be a part of the mix but are usually missing. Estimates are that 80% or more of the body's defense system is in the gut, so the gut flora is intimately involved with overall health. A big part of The Original Diet is devoted to tending to this teeming mass, for unless it is performing properly, illness is likely.

In the alternative health world, there is a great deal of emphasis placed on the use of conventional probiotics, which are supposedly bacterial clones of the "friendly" bacteria that should be in your gut. Taking them in quantity (from 1 billion to 1 trillion) each day will theoretically squeeze out the bad guys, and reestablish a healthy colony. For the purpose of our diet makeover, some may find it helpful to take a probiotic, since gut microbes are intimately involved in the digestive process, and many previously living on the SAD diet are likely to have a mess in their gut. Before we can answer the question of which probiotic to take, if any, we need to step back and look at the big picture.

Based on my research, here is my take on what might be going on in our gut. When we are born our gut is sterile, and we are designed by MA to colonize it from the bacteria in our mother's birth canal on the way out. Well, that moves us to the hospital room, and brings up the following questions: Have the well-meaning staff swabbed the birth canal with anything that might disturb the natural flora? What about the anesthesia or other stuff dripped or injected into the mother – does that affect the natural flora? What about a caesarian section [168]? In the latter instance, we can forget about the birth canal, and assume the baby will colonize his/her gut from a passing nurse, lab technician, or orderly. Not a fun prospect, but wait.

An observation from all of this concerns the general belief that a child can genetically inherit food and other allergies, skin problems, and gastric upsets from their mother. Well, if the gut colonization process works as designed, the baby "inherits" at least some of these characteristics from the birth canal bacteria, which reflects the health (or illnesses) of the mother as reflected by her lifestyle, and is not genetic at all, but it is passed on. So, if you were a C-section baby (possibly itself indicating a less than healthy mother), and the nurse that held you, cleaned you, played with you, and breathed on you was a healthy specimen, you might be way ahead of the game! I can think of a fun animal research project (perhaps it has already been tried) where just before birth, a portion of the mother's birth canal is cleaned of the bacteria in it. It is then replaced with what are hopefully the ideal mix of friendly bacteria to give the offspring a good head start in life, particularly if it is known that the mother has pre-existing health issues.

There is also ample evidence that breast milk is a second source of probiotics from the mother, particularly bifidobacteria for colon colonization, increasing the importance of breast feeding [169]. Along these same lines, we know from anthropological studies that MA's method for human females to give birth is by squatting. I wonder what differences there would be in birth canal probiotic colonization of the child as a result of this position versus the conventional supine position. Certainly, the birth canal would be at a very different angle when squatting, perhaps enhancing colonization.

So, here we are today with a gut full of stuff that has changed over time as a function of just about everything we put into (or even on) our bodies, as well as everything the medical/dental communities put in us. My personal opinion is that if we were to have available to us the gut microbial contents of PA and compare it to anyone now living, there would be few similarities. I would expect to see in the guts of modern humans not only new critters, but also mutated old critters, and this is one reason why I do not think the medical research community will be able to define even a substantial part of our gut contents any time soon, if ever. So far, they have only identified a handful of the hundreds of mutating critters, and by the time they get to the end of that list, hundreds more new ones will have evolved. If my analysis is correct, we actually no longer have a specimen of a healthy gut, so it becomes a guessing game.

In the probiotic industry, they have identified what they believe to be the healthy strains, some of which may be human or animal based, and these are grown using a variety of media (food), including dairy and such esoteric plant products as garbanzo beans. Some require refrigeration and others do not. If the A excludes B theory of new bacteria replacing old were the only thing going on in the gut, perhaps probiotics would always be a good idea, but I do not think it is that simple. I see no reason why Darwin would not be at work in our guts, where survival of the fittest reigns among competing strains and even species. A simple assumption is that they all feed off our bodies, which I am sure many do, but I also would expect to see what are called epiparasites, which are those that feed off other parasites – critter eating critter.

If my assumptions are correct, let's see what might happen if we willy-nilly start taking multi-strain probiotics in large quantities.

Depending on what is waiting at the other end of our esophagus, we may well be sending down food to feed many of the bad guy epiparasites that live off some of these strains, strengthening them and making us sicker. Or, the strains used in the probiotic, for some reason or other, do not match any in our gut, but are close enough so that they can somehow combine with similar strains to create yet a new mutated friend or foe. Please remember that the gut critters we are talking about are not just bacteria, but include the whole gamut of fungi, viruses and various parasites, and it is wishful thinking to assume they do not interact with each other.

Suffice to say that it has been my experience that you can make yourself sicker (or healthier) with probiotics, and it is somewhat of a dice roll [170]. The issues become more complicated for those probiotic supplements that include prebiotics, a food source designed ostensibly to provide nourishment to enhance only the growth of the good guys. Basically, the bad guys may get to it first, and you end up nourishing them. In fact, a recent study of the use of the popular prebiotic known as FOS (fructo-oligosaccharides) in rats found that it actually increased gut permeability (leaky gut), and caused salmonella bacteria to spread outside of the intestines, both of which can contribute to illness [171].

Yet another problem is Small Intestine Bacterial Overgrowth (SIBO). Normally, the stomach and upper portion of the small intestine should be devoid of large colonies of bacteria, but due to improper diet and toxins, the small intestine, in particular, can become host to a variety of bacteria, leading to malabsorption and a host of other symptoms, including IBS (Irritable Bowel Syndrome). There is a simple breath test to determine the presence of SIBO, and the usual treatment is with an antibiotic such as rifaximin [172]. From my research, it appears possible that the bacterial strains normally found in probiotics may end up colonizing in areas where they don't belong [173], another reason not to begin high dose probiotics until diet and detox protocols are in place. Here is my protocol.

It appears that L. acidophilus is a required bacteria strain in the gut, so it should be represented in the product. In addition, B. bifidum and B. longum appear to be somewhat universal, so I limit my intake to those three, and I prefer a human-derived strain, if available, grown on a dairy-free medium. The one I use is Kyo-Dophilus by Wakunaga [174], and I take from one to three per day, with meals. Look for improvement in gut function, such as elimination of gas, diarrhea, and/or constipation, and you may also find some fruit allergies are alleviated [175]. There may be an adjustment period of a few weeks during which some symptoms may be aggravated. Once detoxification has taken place, particularly in the area of parasite cleansing, multi-strain and higher dose protocols might be employed. I believe it is very important also to be taking spore-forming bacteria to complement conventional probiotics.

At this point, I am going to speculate and peer into the future as to the potential impact of the gut microflora on our diet. Gut microflora is a unique bridge between our heritage and our environment. It is a part of our heritage because it is naturally intended to be inherited from our mother at birth. It becomes a part of our environment when it proliferates in our gut, which is outside the body. Finally, it plays a major role in the digestive process. This raises the issue of whether in the future our gut bacteria could be tailored in such a manner that we would be able to digest foods other than those in the Original Diet without ill effect. In other words, perhaps we could bypass the geneticists and accomplish some amount of additional alignment between our heritage and today's environment by fiddling with gut bacteria. Let's see if MA can shed any light on this proposition.

From the discussion of natural toxins in plants, tannins surfaced as a prevalent toxin. A large intake of tannins may cause bowel irritation, kidney irritation, liver damage, irritation of the stomach, and gastrointestinal pain. A correlation has also been made between esophageal cancer in humans and regular consumption of certain foods with high tannin concentrations [176]. Ruminant animals also have difficulty digesting and deriving nutrition from plants with high tannin levels, and hence avoid them unless foods that are more nutritious are not readably available. A research study was conducted in Ethiopia on East African ruminants, including sheep, goats and antelope, where these animals had been found to be eating small amounts of plants with high tannin content, such as the leaves of Acacia trees [177]. Upon examination of the gut bacteria from these animals, they found previously unknown strains, which had the unique property of being able to digest tannins and derive nutrition from them. It is not known how these strains were derived – did they come from long-term ingestion of the Acacia leaves themselves, or did these animals inherit the strains as a biological fluke? In another study, researchers found that they could transplant tannin-digesting bacteria from one mammal (a Hawaiian goat) to another mammal (an Australian goat), who then acquired the ability to safely eat some tannin-containing foods [178].

The upshot from the above studies is the intriguing possibility that similar cultivation and transplanting of gut bacteria in humans may be a way in the not-too-distant future of accelerating the alignment of our evolutionary heritage with today's environment, at least in the area of food digestion. For example, could the transplantation of gut flora from a healthy pie-and-soda-eating *winner* to an *other* convey those same health "benefits" useful in our modern environment?

Gut Repair

Many people have inflamed, angry, and dysfunctional intestines, a likely result of the way they have eaten, the medications they have taken, and their burden of toxicity. This condition is sometimes referred to as chronic gastritis. Each factor undermines the balance of beneficial bacterial flora colonies in the gut lining. If this has taken place, betaine HCl or digestive enzymes might cause some negative reactions such as local pain and headaches. Important elements in gut repair are the fulvic/humic acids and spore-forming bacteria from the diet, which displace some of the bad guys and repopulate with good guys, thus speeding the healing process.

There are several approaches to healing an inflamed (and possibly porous or leaky) gut. One approach uses plant extracts for short-term relief, and the other uses animal products for ultimately healing the lining of the gut. I will discuss the plant extracts first.

Slippery elm bark is a soothing and healing herb for an irritated gut, and can be taken as a tea, powder, or capsule. Large amounts of slippery elm can be taken often, and over time it can help to patch up the gut. Once intestines have healed, HCl and digestive enzymes are more likely to be tolerated. There are many brands on the market, and one can take many grams per day during the healing process, which could take months. Marshmallow root, also widely available, may be used as an alternative to slippery elm bark.

For at least several thousand years, people in the Mediterranean region have used resin from a particular shrub belonging to the Pistachio family for gastrointestinal ailments. The resin is called mastic gum, and it is produced commercially on the Greek island of Chios. Some reports have shown that it has the ability to eliminate the H.pylori bacteria that causes stomach and intestinal ulcers, and it also has anti-fungal properties. Other studies, backed by the pharmaceutical industry, have concluded that it does not reduce H.pylori concentrations, so this is somewhat of a personal trial-and-error process. Like slippery elm, many brands are available and one can take several grams per day.

Notice that the healing supplements in this section use portions of plants that we have eliminated from the Original Diet, like bark, root, and a resin extracted from the bark. This is in keeping with reserving these plant parts for short-term medicinal use, not as nourishment. Depending on one's level of toxicity, none of the above remedies may work. For example, large amounts of mercury can keep the gut in a state of inflammation until sufficient amounts have been removed through detoxification.

Now, let's turn to animal-based gut healing, in the form of gelatin. It was already mentioned in the above discussion of gelatin that it has soothing properties. Like slippery elm and marshmallow root, gelatin also forms a hydrophilic colloid, meaning a water absorbing gel, which coats the intestines and leads to healing. Because gelatin is an integral part of the Original Diet, its long-term use will maintain the integrity of the gut wall.

Last, but by no means least, is clay. Clay is known to adsorb or otherwise render harmless the natural toxins found in foods that you have probably been eating most of your life, and will continue to eat during the diet changeover period. During this diet transition time, sucking on clay tablets between meals during the day may be helpful. One source of clay tablets that I have used is the Terramin brand by California Earth Minerals [179]. I suck on one at a time until it has "dissolved." Swishing the clay around in the mouth is a very good idea (I happen to love the taste of clay). I find that it triggers the thirst response, which may have been long dormant, so I drink lots of water with the clay and avoid taking it with food supplements because it may adsorb them. Many annoying digestive issues may disappear with clay, including food cravings.

Chapter 13 - The Portable Diet

This section is devoted to the busy person who may be on the move a great deal of the time and would like to have a portable version of the Original Diet, so here it is. For animal fat and protein in portable form that requires no refrigeration and will not deteriorate for many months, it is hard to beat pemmican, so I would take along several bars. My favorite is the one from US Original meats [19]. Liver tablets are also a good source of protein and easy to transport. For fruit, I take along fresh fruit. For eggs, I take along hard-boiled eggs. The food supplements are easy to tote except for the red palm oil, which can get somewhat messy. I have been looking for a source of the oil in gelcaps, but have not yet found one. Individual pro-A, vitamin E and vitamin K supplements can be substituted. I do get many stares on the airplane, but a discussion of the Original Diet is sure to break the ice in any conversation!

What happens if I am away from home for some time and cannot get the Original Diet raw materials? Well, my analogy to that is times when, due to environmental disruptions such as long-term drought, PA could not get his/her diet raw materials. To avoid starvation, PA needed to eat items that he/she would normally consider unacceptable. PA was able to manage on a short-term basis by consuming clay with the food, which adsorbed enough of the toxins to enable survival. (Note that adsorption means to form a bond on the surface, as opposed to absorption, which means to diffuse together to form a solution.) So, I add to the portable diet a good supply of clay – don't leave home without it! There are no formal guidelines for this, but taking 1-4 capsules of clay with a "toxic" meal should help matters.

Chapter 14 - Questions Relating to the Diet

I have tried to put on the hat of a reader, and pose questions likely to be asked after reading the diet section.

Isn't the Original Diet like the Atkins diet? The Atkins diet is a low carb diet that allows for: grain-fed as well as commercially-processed meat such as bacon, fried foods, vegetables, dairy, nuts, seeds, artificial sweeteners, fish, fowl, processed oils, and beans such as soy, and does not control the types of liquids. The Original Diet is much more restrictive, disallowing all of the above.

Isn't the Original Diet like the gluten-free/dairy-free diet? The GF/DF diet, as it is known, restricts dairy and gluten-containing grains, but allows other grains, vegetables, juices, nuts, seeds, fish, fowl, grain fed meat, and processed oils, and does not control the types of liquids. The Original Diet is much more restrictive, and perhaps we should call it the SF/DF/VF/SF/NF/RF/OF diet! Did I leave something out?

Isn't the Original Diet like the Paleo diet? There are many so-called Paleo diets out there, but most of them are centered on the late Paleo period after the introduction of cooking, fishing, and bird catching, ignoring the previous 2.4 million years of our heritage. Therefore, they presume that toxic vegetables, nuts, seeds, fish, and fowl were acceptable ancient foods. They also presume that a diet low in saturated fat and salt were standard fare. The result is a diet very different from the Original Diet.

Can't I have a bagel with cream cheese just once a week? Nobody is perfect, so if you "cheat," take some clay with the meal. Closely monitor how you feel afterward to see if you can detect any negative effects.

I am healthy, so why should I consider the Original Diet? Perhaps you shouldn't consider it. Here is one plan that you might follow. If you believe you are in a good state of health, there may be no reason to modify any of your food choices at all. If you are the self-experimenting type and/or are interested in illness prevention, you could try various combinations of the Tier One, Two, and Three food choices, knowing the relative toxin issues relating to each. If you are suffering from health issues, you might want to gravitate to the Tier One Original Diet, beginning as slowly as you wish, to see if you notice improvements.

If I follow the Original Diet, will my [insert symptom or illness] go away? The only way I know to answer this question would be to try the diet. Please remember that to achieve overall health, detox (consult *The Wellness Project*) may be just as important as, or more important than diet. Because everyone's health history is different, I do not believe it is possible to predict the degree of success that can be achieved.

What do you think of [insert name of supplement or treatment]? As a researcher, I am very open to reviewing what others are doing in the health field, and I have been doing so for decades. The Original Diet is a distillation of this research in the area of nutrition, and contains what I currently believe to be the essentials for a healthy diet. I am no longer a supplement junkie, and try to minimize using anything that was not available to PA. I fully intent to continue my research and to discuss any updated findings at www.theoriginofhealth.com.   Because we have become accustomed to the take-a-pill-feel-better approach of big pharma, I have seen many people pick and choose among supplements in an effort to get a quick fix (I used to do it, too). The Original Diet does not work that way, and piecemeal supplementation may provide unpredictable or no positive effects.

The Original Diet and all the supplements are expensive, so what should I do if I can't afford it? It is certainly true that organic grass-fed meat and organically grown fruit are more expensive than macaroni and cheese, and some of the supplements I suggest are pricey. Illness is also expensive, in terms of treatment, loss of work, and the impact on one's lifestyle. Each person must make a choice regarding the use of his or her financial resources. It would be great if, instead of subsidizing "health" care (it is really *illness* care), the government offered to subsidize illness prevention, but it is doubtful that we will see such a shift in our lifetime.

What do *you* eat on a typical day? First, bear in mind that I eat the purist, Tier One, version of the diet, primarily because I feel better when I do, and I like to self-experiment. Of course, I cheat occasionally, keeping my clay nearby. I do not expect many others to follow Tier One as closely as I, unless they are motivated to do so by some health issues. For breakfast, I might have a baked organic-grass-fed free-range rib-eye steak with a half-grapefruit and some hot fruit tea made with mineral-rich water. I use plenty of salt on the steak and grapefruit. If I want a morning snack, it might be one or two lightly boiled high omega-3 egg yolks and a green apple, perhaps with some desiccated liver. I drink a glass of mineral-rich water between meals. For lunch, a baked ground-buffalo burger, salted, with a bowl of blueberries, and some hot water or fruit tea.

If I want an afternoon snack, pemmican and a slice of melon are good choices. I drink another glass of mineral-rich water between meals. For dinner, I might have a couple of baked organic-grass-fed loin lamb chops, or perhaps baby-back pork ribs, salted, with some pineapple, and bone-stock soup. I avoid eating after dinner, but drink more mineral-rich water. All of the animal foods are cooked in glass dishes in a convection oven. I take the food supplements mentioned above, including liver, glandulars, and red palm oil. As a reminder, Appendix B is a chart summarizing the diet, including supplements. Appendix C is a list of resources for obtaining the various foods and supplements used in the diet.

Section Five - The Future

The significant problems we have cannot be solved at the
same level of thinking with which we created them. –
Albert Einstein

The purpose of this section is to summarize a few areas of future research that I believe will be most beneficial to the health of our population (and humans in general). The first area is that of nutritional research. I'm referring to studies such as those that purportedly show saturated fat contributes to heart disease; that salt is a cause of high blood pressure; that eating according to the FDA pyramid will make you healthy; or that following any of the dietary guidelines put out by diabetes, heart, or cancer societies will in any way provide a health benefit.

My suggestion is that in the future, for the sake of accuracy, peer-reviewed journals should, for all nutrition study participants, publish a list of all of the foods they were and are eating. This should include the source of those foods (e.g. was the meat grain-fed, and were all foods organic or GMO) along with an inventory of all known toxins in the body of study participants, such as a count of each person's amalgams and root canals, and a list of all medications taken and being taken during the study. Because of its unique importance, magnesium levels should also be tested and reported in any study having to do with cardiovascular issues. In other words, the objective is to establish a baseline control for these studies, just as we have established a baseline diet. To do otherwise is just inadequate science. Of course, what I would ideally like to see are existing studies repeated with participants that have followed The Original Diet for some time, to see what the difference would be in outcome. It is unlikely that any commercial enterprise would fund such studies because, not only is there no money in it, the results could very well dramatically curtail existing sales of drugs and supplements. So private funding is the only alternative.

In the fruit arena, efforts should be made to halt any genetic modifications to fruit-bearing plants, since the effects on humans are unknown, and the potential for harm is enormous.

In the dirt arena, I believe that research into the missing components of our diet from soil, including humic and fulvic acids and soil bacteria such as the spore-formers, could produce dramatic health benefits for virtually all categories of illness. In a broader sense, such a study should also encompass the study of gut bacteria as it applies to health.

I realize that several of the protocols disclosed in this book are not easy to implement, due to a variety of factors such as availability of products, space limitations, and a general reluctance to make radical lifestyle modifications. Therefore, I propose the establishment of neighborhood wellness centers where many of the diet protocols of The Original Diet and the detox protocols of *The Wellness Project* would be made available to the public. A patent application has been filed covering this concept.

It is my intention to devote a portion of the profits from the sale of this book and the licensing of my inventions in the health field to research efforts such as those described above, and I hope there are some readers who will share my passion.

Lastly, I would like to propose a new paradigm for the relationship between a prospective patient and an internist or family doctor. I believe that such a relationship should always begin with the following queries by the doctor:

➢   Provide a one-week diary of everything you put into or on your body, where the entries are made in real time (record the information when you are ingesting or applying the item). Include how food is cooked, what kind of containers are used, and brand names of products. Be sure to include all medications, supplements, cleansers, and cosmetics.

➢   Provide a one-week diary of everything that comes out of your body, including frequency of urinations and their color and odor; stool frequency and description; and sweat odor.

➢   Describe your environment – whether mostly indoor or outdoor, age and construction of house, use of carpeting, water supply and filtration, air filtration, use of spas and pools, and use of pesticides.

➢ Provide complete dental records, including the placement of restorations, materials used, and dates of placement. List all root-canalled teeth, and the age of them.

In addition, I believe the prospective patient is entitled to request from the doctor a list of all of the medications the doctor is taking. The objective is to enable the patient to determine if the side-effect profile of any of these medications might impair the doctor's ability to perform.

As a final note, it is my intention to continue my research into The Original Diet and generate periodic updates to the information in this book. A website is under construction to facilitate communication with readers, and it will appear at *www.theoriginofhealth.com*.

Appendix A

Publications

➢ NASA Tech Brief Document ID: 19660000034 Valve Driver Circuits

➢ NASA Tech Brief – Triple Redundant Spacecraft Attitude Control System

➢ NASA Tech Report #JPL-TR-32-1011. DIANA – A Digital-Analog Simulation Program

➢ NASA Tech Report Document ID: 19680052463 Attitude Control of an Electrically Propelled Spacecraft Utilizing the Primary Thrust System

➢ NASA Tech Report #JPL-TR-32-1104. The Analysis and Configuration of a Control System for a Mars Propulsive Lander

➢ NASA Tech Report Document ID: 19670060448. Computer Analysis and Simulation of Mars Soft Landing Descent Control System Combining Inertial and Radar Sensing Techniques

➢ NASA Tech Report Document ID: 19670006377. Propulsive Planetary Landing Capsule Control System

➢ NASA Tech Report Document ID: 19670005459 Sterilization of Guidance and Control Systems and Components

➢ The Analysis and Configuration of a Control System for a Mars Propulsive Lander (Computer analysis and simulation of Mars soft landing descent control system combining inertial and radar sensing techniques) Mankovitz, R J, International Federation Of Automatic Control, Symposium On Automatic Control In Space, 2nd, Vienna, Austria; 4-8 Sept. 1967. P. 21.

➢ MIL-R-28750 Solid State Relay Military Specification

➢ EIA RS-433 Solid State Relay Standards

➢ Author of "THE LAW," a monthly column in Electronic Engineering Times discussing intellectual property law.

AFFILIATIONS   Intellectual Property Section- CA State Bar

AND HONORS: Eta Kappa Nu- Engineering Honor Society

                     Who's Who in California – 1983

Patents

(Health related patents are in **bold**):

PAT. #	Title
6,987,842	Electronic television program guide delivery system using telephone network idle time
RE38,600	Apparatus and methods for accessing information relating to radio television programs
6,783,754	**Plant-based non-toxic sunscreen products**
6,760,537	Apparatus and method for television program scheduling
6,701,060	Enhancing operations of video tape cassette players
6,687,906	EPG with advertising inserts
6,606,747	System and method for grazing television channels from an electronic program guide
6,549,719	Television program record scheduling and satellite receiver control using compressed codes
6,487,362	Enhancing operations of video tape cassette recorders
6,477,705	Method and apparatus for transmitting, storing, and processing electronic program guide data for on-screen display
6,441,862	Combination of VCR index and EPG
6,361,397	**Garments which facilitate the drainage of lymphatic fluid from the breast area of the human female**
6,341,195	Apparatus and methods for a television on-screen guide
6,321,381	Apparatus and method for improved parental control of television use
6,253,069	Methods and apparatus for providing information in response to telephonic requests
6,239,794	Method and system for simultaneously displaying a television program and information about the program

RE37,131   Apparatus and methods for music and lyrics broadcasting

6,154,203   System and method for grazing television channels from an electronic
program guide

6,147,715   Combination of VCR index and EPG

6,125,231   Method of adding titles to a directory of television programs recorded on a
video tape

6,122,011   Apparatus and method for creating or editing a channel map

6,117,050   Exercise apparatus for use with conventional chairs

6,115,057   Apparatus and method for allowing rating level control of the viewing of a
program

6,091,884   Enhancing operations of video tape cassette players

**6,086,450   Brassieres which facilitate the drainage of lymphatic fluid from the breast
area of the human female**

6,072,520   System for improved parental control of television use

6,028,599   Database for use in method and apparatus for displaying television
programs and related text

6,010,430   Exercise apparatus for use with conventional chairs

5,995,092   Television system and method for subscription of information services

5,987,213   System and method for automatically recording television programs in
television systems with tuners external to video recorders

5,949,492   Apparatus and methods for accessing information relating to radio
television programs

5,949,471   Apparatus and method for improved parental control of television use

5,921,900   Exercise apparatus for use with conventional chairs

5,915,026   System and method for programming electronic devices from a remote site

5,734,786   Apparatus and methods for deriving a television guide from audio signals

5,703,795   Apparatus and methods for accessing information relating to radio and
            television programs

5,690,594   Exercise apparatus for use with conventional chairs

5,677,895   Apparatus and methods for setting timepieces

5,640,484   Switch for automatic selection of television signal sources for delivery of
            television guide data

5,633,918   Information distribution system

5,581,614   Method for encrypting and embedding information in a video program

5,577,108   Information distribution system with self-contained programmable
            automatic interface unit

5,561,849   Apparatus and method for music and lyrics broadcasting

5,559,550   Apparatus and methods for synchronizing a clock to a network clock

5,552,837   Remote controller for scanning data and controlling a video system

5,543,929   Television for controlling a video cassette recorder to access programs on a
            video cassette tape

5,541,738   Electronic program guide

5,526,284   Apparatus and methods for music and lyrics broadcasting

5,523,794   Method and apparatus for portable storage and use of data transmitted by
            television signal

5,515,173   System and method for automatically recording television programs in
            television systems with tuners external to video recorders

5,512,963   Apparatus and methods for providing combining multiple video sources

5,499,103   Apparatus for an electronic guide with video clips

5,465,240   Apparatus and methods for displaying text in conjunction with recorded
            audio programs

5,408,686   Apparatus and methods for music and lyrics broadcasting

5,385,733   **Topical preparation and method for suppression of skin eruptions caused by herpes simplex virus**

5,382,983   Apparatus and method for total parental control of television use

5,215,748   **Topical preparation and method for suppression of skin eruptions caused herpes simplex virus**

5,161,251   Apparatus and methods for providing text information identifying audio program selections

5,159,191   Apparatus and method for using ambient light to control electronic apparatus

5,134,719   Apparatus and methods for identifying broadcast audio program selections in an FM stereo broadcast system

5,119,507   Receiver apparatus and methods for identifying broadcast audio program selections in a radio broadcast system

5,119,503   Apparatus and methods for broadcasting auxiliary data in an FM stereo broadcast system

3,691,426   Current Limiter Responsive to Current Flow and Temperature Rise

3,648,075   Zero Voltage Switching AC Relay Circuit

Some health related pending patent applications

Food Compositions and Methods

A Method Of Providing An Eating Plan Having A Very Low Concentration Of Natural Toxins

Silver/Plastic Combination that Binds Hazardous Agents and Provides Anti-Microbial Protection

Iodine Containing Compositions

Systems and Methods for Electrically Grounding Humans to Enhance Detoxification

Apparatus and Methods for Reducing Exposure to RF Energy Produced by Portable Transmitters

Soil Based Composition and Method for Removal of Toxins from Mammals

Methods of Providing to the Public Healthy Diet, Detoxification and Lifestyle Protocols in the Form of Neighborhood Centers

Appendix B - Food and Supplement Schedule

TIME	DIET

Awakening
 	
&
 	
Bedtime
	Mineral Water – 10 oz
	Dolomite – 1 tablet
	   Optional: HCl Plus – 1 tab
	Optional per magnesium test:
	   Magnesium taurate -
	      1 cap or tab
	
	Fulvic/Humic acid – 1 capsule/AM
	Spore-formers – 1 capsule/AM
	ProBoost – 1 packet/PM
	Sublingual P5P – 2 tablets

Breakfast
 	
&
 	
Lunch
 	
&
 	
Dinner
	Animal Foods
	Fruit
	Salt
	Hot Water or Fruit Tea – 8 oz
	Red Palm Oil – 1 tsp
	 (or: vit. E, K, carotenoids/AM)
	Eggs (optional)
	Vitamin C – 500 mg
	Desiccated Liver – 5 tablets/1 tsp
	Vitamin D3 – per test results
	      (or UV light)
	Multimineral – 1 capsule
	Gelatin – 1 Tsp./Bone Broth
	Probiotic – 1 capsule
	Glandular – 2 tablets
	Optional:
	  Digestive Enzymes
	  Betaine HCl
	  Bile Salts
	  Pantethine – 300 mg
	  Vitamin B-5 - 500 mg

Between Breakfast and Lunch
 	
&
 	
Between Lunch and Dinner
	Mineral Water – 16 oz
	   Dolomite 1 tablet
	   Vitamin C 500 mg
	         Optional: HCl Plus – 1 tab
	   Optional per magnesium test:
	   Magnesium taurate –
	      1 cap or tab
	Gut Repair as necessary

Appendix C - Food and Supplement Resources

(see www.theoriginofhealth.com for a list of website links)

Food or Supplement	Resource	Website
Animal Foods	Local health food stores or farmers' markets; US Original Meats; North Star Bison; Blackwing Ostrich	www.uswellnessmeats.com www.northstarbison.com www.blackwing.com
Fruits	Local health food stores or farmers' markets; Brownwood Acres fruit supplements	www.brownwoodacres.com
Eggs	Local health food stores or farmers' markets – look for high omega-3 feed; Example: Christopher Eggs	www.christophereggs.com
Salt	RealSalt	www.realsalt.com
Glandulars; Vitamin A; Vitamin D; HCl Plus	Neonatal Glandular; Bio-Ae-Mulsion; Bio-D-Mulsion; HCl Plus by Biotics Research	www.bioticsresearch.com
Apple Pectin; Betaine HCL; Potassium citrate	Apple Pectin USP; Betaine HCL with pepsin; Potassium Citrate by Twinlab	www.twinlab.com
Water filters	Doulton Water Filters; WellnessFilters	www.doulton.ca www.wellnessfilter.com
Dolomite; Vitamin C	Dolomite 44 grain; Vitamin C 500 mg by Nature's Plus	www.naturesplus.com
Probiotic	Kyo-Dophilus by Wakunaga	www.kyolic.com
Humic/Fulvic Acids	Immune Boost 77 (capsules) and Vitality Boost HA by MorningStar Minerals; Metal Magnet by PhytoPharmica	www.msminerals.com www.phytopharmica.com
Spore-formers	Flora Balance by O'Donnell Formulas; Lactobacillus Sporongenes by Thorne and Pure Encapsulations	www.flora-balance.com www.thorne.com www.purecaps.com
Edible Clay	Pascalite; Terramin; Redmond Clay	www.pascalite.com www.terrapond.com www.redmondclay.com
Multimineral	Citramin II by Thorne Research	www.thorne.com
Vit K complex; Vit E complex	Super K; Gamma E Tocopherol/Tocotrienols; by Life Extension Foundation	www.lef.org

Liver tablets and powder; Slippery Elm Bromelain	Liver; Slippery Elm Bark Powder; Bromelain by NOW Foods	www.nowfoods.com
Red Palm Oil	Tropical Traditions Organic	www.tropicaltraditions.com
Gelatin	Beef Gelatin By Great Lakes Gelatin	www.greatlakesgelatin.com
Magnesium taurate	Magnesium Taurate caps by Cardiovascular Research; Magnesium Taurate 400 tabs by Douglas Labs	www.douglaslabs.com
Magnesium Lotion and bath crystals	Dr. Shealy's Biogenics Magnesium Lotion; Magnesium Chloride Crystals	www.selfhealthsystems.com
Zinc Lotion	Zinc Sulphate Lotion by Kirkman Labs	www.kirkmanlabs.com
Sublingual B-6; Sublingual B Complex; Zinc; SAMe; Mastic Gum	Coenzymated B-6, sublingual; Coenzymated B Complex; OptiZinc; SAMe; Mastic Gum capsules By Source Naturals	www.sourcenaturals.com
Bile Salts	Cholacol by Standard Process; or Beta Plus by Biotics Research	www.standardprocess.com www.bioticsresearch.com
Water Bottles	Glass bottles by ebottle.com	www.ebottle.com
EXATEST	EXATEST by IntraCellular Diagnostics	www.exatest.com

Bibliography

1. Mankovitz, R., *The Wellness Project - A Rocket Scientist's Blueprint for Health*. 2008, Santa Barbara: Montecito Wellness LLC. 360 pp.
2. Mankovitz, R., *Nature's Detox Plan - A Program for Physical and Emotional Detoxification*. 2008, Santa Barbara: Montecito Wellness LLC. 196 pp.
3. Gershon, M.D., *The Second Brain: A Groundbreaking New Understanding of Nervous Disorders of the Stomach and Intestine*. 1999: HarperPerennial.
4. Cohen, M.N. and G.J. Armelagos, *Paleopathology at the Origins ofAgriculture*. 1984: New York: Academic Press.
5. Diamond, J., *The Worst Mistake in the History of the Human Race*. Discover, 1987. 8(5): p. 64-66.
6. Price, W.A., *Nutrition and Physical Degeneration: A Comparison of Primitive and Modern Diets and Their Effects*. 1970: Price-Pottenger Foundation.
7. www.westonaprice.org, *Weston A. Price Foundation*
8. Engel, C., *Wild Health: How Animals Keep Themselves Well and What We Can Learn from Them*. 2002: Houghton Mifflin.
9. Cordain, L., *The Paleo diet*. 2002: Wiley.
10. Pottenger, E., *Pottenger's Cats: A Study in Nutrition (edited writings of Francis Pottenger)*. La Mesa, California: The Price-Pottenger Nutrition Foundation, 1983.
11. www.paleodiet.com, *Paleolithic Diet Page*
12. Diamond, J., *The Third Chimpanzee*. 1993, New York: HarperCollins.
13. www.ppnf.org, *Price-Pottenger Nutrition Foundation*
14. www.northstarbison.com, *Grassfed American Bison*
15. www.blackwing.com, *Blackwing Ostrich Meat*
16. Lame Deer, J. and R. Erdoes, *Lame Deer, Seeker of Visions*. 1972: Simon and Schuster.
17. Fallon, S., P. Connolly, and M.G. Enig, *Nourishing Traditions: The Cookbook that Challenges Politically Correct Nutrition and the Diet Dictocrats*. 1999: NewTrends Pub.

18.   Anderson, A.K., H.E. Gayley, and A.D. Pratt, *Studies on the Chemical Composition of Bovine Blood.* Journal of Dairy Science, 1930. **13**(4): p. 336.

19.   www.uswellnessmeats.com, *U.S. Wellness Meats*

20.   www.lifelinescreening.com, *Life Line Screening*

21.   www.thincs.org, *The International Network of Cholesterol Skeptics*

22.   Kauffman, J.M., *Misleading Recent Papers on Statin Drugs in Peer-Reviewed Medical Journals.* Journal of American Physicians and Surgeons Volume, 2007. **12**(1): p. 7.

23.   Kauffman, J.M., *Malignant Medical Myths.* 2006: Infinity Publishing.

24.   Graveline, D., *Thief of Memory: Statin Drugs and the Misguided War on Cholesterol.* 2004: Infinity Publishing, Havenford, PA.

25.   Seelig, M.S. and A. Rosanoff, *The Magnesium Factor.* 2003: Avery.

26.   Dean, C., *The Miracle of Magnesium.* 2003: Ballantine Books.

27.   Purvis, J.R. and A. Movahed, *Magnesium disorders and cardiovascular diseases.* Clin Cardiol, 1992. **15**(8): p. 556-68.

28.   Rosanoff, A. and M.S. Seelig, *Comparison of Mechanism and Functional Effects of Magnesium and Statin Pharmaceuticals.* Journal of the American College of Nutrition, 2004. **23**(5): p. 501-505.

29.   Leopold, A.C. and R. Ardrey, *Toxic Substances in Plants and the Food Habits of Early Man.* Science, 1972. **176**(4034): p. 512-514.

30.   Whittaker, R.H. and P.P. Feeny, *Allelochemics: Chemical Interactions between Species.* Science, 1971. **171**(3973): p. 757-770.

31.   Liener, I., *Toxic constituents of plant foodstuffs.* 1980, New York: Academic Press.

32.   NRC, *Lost Crops of Africa: Volume III: Fruits.* 2008, Washington DC: National Academies Press.

33.   Peters, C.R., E.M. O'Brien, and R.B. Drummond, *Edible Wild Plants of Sub-Saharan Africa.* Royal Botanical Gardens, Kew, 1992.

34.   Baker, L.C., L.H. Lampitt, and O.B. Meredith, *Solanine glycoside of the potato III. An improved method of extraction and determination.* J. Sci. Food and Agric, 1955. **6**: p. 197-202.

35.   Sizer, C.E., J.A. Maga, and C.J. Craven, *Total glycoalkaloids in potatoes and potato chips*. Journal of Agricultural and Food Chemistry, 1980. **28**(3): p. 578-579.

36.   Rayburn, J.R., J.A. Bantle, and M. Friedman, *Role of Carbohydrate Side Chains of Potato Glycoalkaloids in Developmental Toxicity*. Journal of Agricultural and Food Chemistry, 1994. **42**(7): p. 1511-1515.

37.   Lachman, J., et al., *Potato Glycoalkaloids and their significance in plant protection and human nutrition–Review*. Czechoslovkia, Series Rostlinna Vyroba, 2001. **47**(4): p. 181-191.

38.   Johns, T., *Detoxification function of geophagy and domestication of the potato*. Journal of Chemical Ecology, 1986. **12**(3): p. 635-646.

39.   Dashwood, R.H., *Indole-3-carbinol: Anticarcinogen or tumor promoter in brassica vegetables?* Chemico-Biological Interactions, 1998. **110**(1-2): p. 1-5.

40.   Park, J., M. Shigenaga, and B. Ames, *Induction of cytochrome P4501A1 by 2, 3, 7, 8-tetrachlorodibenzo-p-dioxin or indolo (3, 2-b) carbazole is associated with oxidative DNA damage*. Proc Natl Acad Sci US A, 1996. **93**(6): p. 2322-2327.

41.   Altmann, S.A., S.L. Garrigues, and A.B. Stahl, *More on Hominid Diet Before Fire*. Current Anthropology, 1985. **26**(5): p. 661-663.

42.   Blumenschine, R.J., A. Whiten, and K. Hawkes, *Hominid Carnivory and Foraging Strategies, and the Socio-Economic Function of Early Archaeological Sites [and Discussion]*. Philosophical Transactions: Biological Sciences, 1991. **334**(1270): p. 211-221.

43.   Luchterhand, K., *On Early Hominid Plant-Food Niches*. Current Anthropology, 1982. **23**(2): p. 211-218.

44.   Peters, C.R., et al., *The Early Hominid Plant-Food Niche: Insights From an Analysis of Plant Exploitation by Homo, Pan, and Papio in Eastern and Southern Africa [and Comments and Reply]*. Current Anthropology, 1981. **22**(2): p. 127-140.

45.   Stahl, A.B., et al., *Hominid Dietary Selection Before Fire [and Comments and Reply]*. Current Anthropology, 1984. **25**(2): p. 151-168.

46.   Milton, K., *Nutritional characteristics of wild primate foods: do the diets of our closest living relatives have lessons for us?* Nutrition, 1999. **15**(6): p. 488-498.

47.   Seelig, M.S., *Epidemiology of water magnesium; evidence of contributions to health.* The Magnesium Web Site.

48.   Durlach, J., M. Bara, and A. Guiet-Bara, *Magnesium level in drinking water: its importance in cardiovascular risk.* Magnesium in Health and Disease, 1989: p. 173-182.

49.   www.mgwater.com, *The Magnesium Web Site*

50.   www.ntllabs.com, *Water Testing: National Testing Labs*

51.   www.naturesplus.com, *.: Nature's Plus*

52.   Rodale, J.I. and H.J. Taub, *Magnesium, the Nutrient that Could Change Your Life.* 1968: Pyramid Books.

53.   Kok, F.J., et al., *SERUM COPPER AND ZINC AND THE RISK OF DEATH FROM CANCER AND CARDIOVASCULAR DISEASE.* American Journal of Epidemiology, 2002. **128**(2): p. 352-359.

54.   www.doulton.ca, *Doulton Water Filters*

55.   www.wellnessfilter.com, *Wellness Filters*

56.   Shotyk, W., M. Krachler, and B. Chen, *Contamination of Canadian and European bottled waters with antimony from PET containers.* Journal of Environmental Monitoring, 2006. **8**(2): p. 288-292.

57.   Robbins, W.J. and A. Hervey, *Toxicity of Water Stored in Polyethylene Bottles.* Bulletin of the Torrey Botanical Club, 1974. **101**(5): p. 287-291.

58.   Le, H.H., et al., *Bisphenol A is released from polycarbonate drinking bottles and mimics the neurotoxic actions of estrogen in developing cerebellar neurons.* Toxicology Letters, 2008. **176**(2): p. 149-156.

59.   www.ebottle.com, *Glass Bottles*

60.   www.humichealth.info, *HumicHealth.info*

61.   Fung-Jou Lu, H.-P.H.H.Y.Y.Y., *Fluorescent humic substances- arsenic complex in well water in areas where blackfoot disease is endemic in Taiwan.* APPLIED ORGANOMETALLIC CHEMISTRY, 1991. 5(6): p. 507-512.

62.   www.humates.com, *Mesa Verde Resources - Humate Supplier*

63.   www.hagroup.neu.edu, *NEU Humic Acid Research Group*

64.   www.msminerals.com, *Morningstar Minerals*

65.   Huynh A Hong , L.H.D., Simon M Cutting *The use of bacterial spore formers as probiotics.* FEMS Microbiol Rev, 2005. **29**(4): p. 813-35.

66.   Ricca, E., A.O. Henriques, and S.M. Cutting, *Bacterial spore formers: probiotics and emerging applications.* 2004: Horizon Bioscience Wymondham, UK.

67.   De Oliveira, E.J., et al., *Molecular Characterization of Brevibacillus laterosporus and Its Potential Use in Biological Control.* Applied and Environmental Microbiology, 2004. **70**(11): p. 6657-6664.

68.   www.thorne.com, *Thorne Research, Inc.*

69.   www.purecaps.com, *Pure Encapsulations*

70.   Corsello, S., MD, *Bacillus Laterosporus BOD.* 1996, New York: Healing Wisdom.

71.   www.flora-balance.com, *Flora Balance: Bacillus Laterosporus*

72.   Stefansson, V., *The Fat of the Land.* 1956: Macmillan.

73.   www.celestialpets.com, *Celestial Pets*

74.   Eriksson, P., C. Fischer, and A. Fredriksson, *Polybrominated Diphenyl Ethers, A Group of Brominated Flame Retardants, Can Interact with Polychlorinated Biphenyls in Enhancing Developmental Neurobehavioral Defects.* Toxicological Sciences, 2006. **94**(2): p. 302.

75.   Enser, M., et al., *The polyunsaturated fatty acid composition of beef and lamb liver.* Meat Science, 1998. **49**(3): p. 321-327.

76.   www.vitalchoice.com, *Vital Choice Wild Seafood*

77.   Nakajima, Y., et al., *Ingestion of Hijiki seaweed and risk of arsenic poisoning.* APPLIED ORGANOMETALLIC CHEMISTRY, 2006. **20**(9): p. 557.

78.   www.diagnostechs.com, *Diagnostechs, Inc.*

79.   www.realmilk.com, *A CAMPAIGN FOR RAW) MILK*

80.   Mandavgane, S.A., V.V. Pattalwar, and A.R. Kalambe, *Development of cow dung based herbal mosquito repellent.* Natural Product Radiance, 2005. **4**(4): p. 270-272.

81.   Campbell, T.C., *The China Study.* 2005: BenBella Books, Dallas.

82.   Bohn, T., et al., *Phytic acid added to white-wheat bread inhibits fractional apparent magnesium absorption in humans.* American Journal of Clinical Nutrition, 2004. **79**(3): p. 418-423.

83.   Duncan, C.W., C.C. Lightfoot, and C.F. Huffman, *Studies on the Composition of Bovine Blood: I. The Magnesium Content of the*

Blood Plasma of the Normal Dairy Calf. J. Dairy Sci., 1938.
21(11): p. 689-696.

84. Odvina, C.V., et al., *Severely Suppressed Bone Turnover: A Potential Complication of Alendronate Therapy.* 2005, Endocrine Soc. p. 1294-1301.

85. Ruggiero, S.L., et al., *Osteonecrosis of the jaws associated with the use of bisphosphonates: a review of 63 cases.* Journal of Oral and Maxillofacial Surgery, 2004. **62**(5): p. 527-534.

86. Sabrina C. Agarwal, M.D.G., *Bone quantity and quality in past populations.* The Anatomical Record, 1996. **246**(4): p. 423-432.

87. Bischoff-Ferrari, H.A., et al., *Calcium intake and hip fracture risk in men and women: a meta-analysis of prospective cohort studies and randomized controlled trials.* American Journal of Clinical Nutrition, 2007. **86**(6): p. 1780.

88. www.breastpumpsdirect.com, *Electric Breast Pumps*

89. www.llli.org, *La Leche League International*

90. Alvarez, H.P., *Grandmother hypothesis and primate life histories.* AMERICAN JOURNAL OF PHYSICAL ANTHROPOLOGY, 2000. **113**(3): p. 435-450.

91. Martin, M.C., et al., *Menopause without symptoms: the endocrinology of menopause among rural Mayan Indians.* Am J Obstet Gynecol, 1993. **168**(6 Pt 1): p. 1839-45.

92. Stewart, D.E., *Menopause in highland Guatemala Mayan women.* Maturitas, 2003. **44**(4): p. 293-7.

93. Lock, M., *Menopause: lessons from anthropology.* 1998, Am Psychosomatic Soc. p. 410-419.

94. www.bioticsresearch.com, *Biotics Research*

95. Cronin, C.C. and F. Shanahan, *Why is celiac disease so common in Ireland.* Perspect Biol Med, 2001. **44**(3): p. 342-52.

96. Gotthoffer, N.R., *Gelatin in nutrition and medicine.* 1945.

97. Daniel, K.T., *The Whole Soy Story: The Dark Side of America's Favorite Health Food.* 2005: New Trends Publishing.

98. Finley, J.W., et al., *Bioavailability of selenium from meat and broccoli as determined by retention and distribution of 75 Se.* Biological Trace Element Research, 2004. **99**(1): p. 191-209.

99. Zheng, J.J., et al., *Measurement of zinc bioavailability from beef and a ready-to-eat high-fiber breakfast cereal in humans:*

application of a whole-gut lavage technique. Am J Clin Nutr, 1993. **58**(6): p. 902-7.

100.   Schuiling, M. and H.C. Harries, *The coconut palm in East Africa.* East African Tall. Principes, 1994. **38**(1): p. 4-11.

101.   Petroianu, G.A., *Green coconut water for intravenous use: Trace and minor element content.* The Journal of Trace Elements in Experimental Medicine, 2004. **17**(4): p. 273-282.

102.   Mercola, J., *Sweet Deception: Why Splenda, NutraSweet, and the FDA May Be Hazardous to Your Health.* 2006: Nelson Books.

103.   Ming, D. and G. Hellekant, *Brazzein, a new high-potency thermostable sweet protein from Pentadiplandra brazzeana B.* FEBS Lett, 1994. **355**(1): p. 106-8.

104.   Parke, D.V. and A.L. Parke, *Rapeseed oil: An autoxidative food lipid.* Journal of clinical biochemistry and nutrition, 1999. **26**(2): p. 51-61.

105.   www.brownwoodacres.com, *Brownwood Acres Fruit Supplements*

106.   Hirsch, J., et al., *Indicators of Erythrocyte Damage after Microwave Warming of Packed Red Blood Cells.* Clin Chem, 2003. **49**(5): p. 792-799.

107.   Lubec, G., C. Wolf, and B. Bartosch, *Aminoacid isomerisation and microwave exposure.* Lancet, 1989. **2**(8676): p. 1392-3.

108.   Arvanitoyannis, I. and L. Bosnea, *Migration of Substances from Food Packaging Materials to Foods.* Critical Reviews in Food Science and Nutrition, 2004. **44**(2): p. 63-76.

109.   Said, Z.M., et al., *Pyridoxine uptake by colonocytes: A specific and regulated carrier-mediated process.* Am J Physiol Cell Physiol, 2008: p. 00015.2008.

110.   Ershoff, B.H., *Protective Effects of Liver in Immature Rats Fed Toxic Doses of Thiouracil.* Journal of Nutrition, 1954. **52**(3): p. 437.

111.   Ershoff, B.H., *Increased Survival of Liver-Fed Rats Administered Multiple Sublethal Doses of X-Irradiation.* Journal of Nutrition, 1952. **47**(2): p. 289.

112.   www.nowfoods.com, *NOW Foods*

113.   Leklem, J.E. and C.B. Hollenbeck, *Acute ingestion of glucose decreases plasma pyridoxal 5'-phosphate and total vitamin B-6 concentration.* Am J Clin Nutr, 1990. **51**(5): p. 832-6.

114.   Wei, I.L., Y.H. Huang, and G.S. Wang, *Vitamin B6 deficiency decreases the glucose utilization in cognitive brain structures of rats.* The Journal of Nutritional Biochemistry, 1999. **10**(9): p. 525-531.

115.   www.sourcenaturals.com, *Source Naturals*

116.   www.tropicaltraditions.com, *Tropical Traditions - Palm Oil*

117.   www.palmoilworld.org, *Palm Oil World*

118.   www.jarrow.com, *Jarrow Formulas*

119.   www.lef.org, *Life Extension Foundation*

120.   Holick, M.F. and M. Jenkins, *The UV Advantage.* 2004: Simon & Schuster.

121.   www.vitamindcouncil.com, *Vitamin D Council*

122.   Binkley, N., et al., *Low Vitamin D Status despite Abundant Sun Exposure.* Journal of Clinical Endocrinology & Metabolism, 2007. **92**(6): p. 2130.

123.   Bastuji-Garin, S. and T.L. Diepgen, *Cutaneous malignant melanoma, sun exposure, and sunscreen use: epidemiological evidence.* British Journal of Dermatology, 2002. **146**(s61): p. 24-30.

124.   Elwood, J.M., *Melanoma and sun exposure: An overview of published studies.* International Journal of Cancer, 1997. **73**(2): p. 198-203.

125.   Whang, R., D.D. Whang, and M.P. Ryan, *Refractory potassium repletion. A consequence of magnesium deficiency.* Archives of Internal Medicine, 1992. **152**(1): p. 40-45.

126.   Seelig, M.S., *Consequences of magnesium deficiency on the enhancement of stress reactions; preventive and therapeutic implications (a review).* 1994, Am Coll Nutrition. p. 429-446.

127.   Gontijo-Amaral, C., et al., *Oral magnesium supplementation in asthmatic children: a double-blind randomized placebo-controlled trial.* Eur J Clin Nutr, 2006. **61**: p. 54–60.

128.   www.magnesiumresearchlab.com, *Magnesium Research Lab*

129.   Arnold, A., et al., *Magnesium deficiency in critically ill patients.* Anaesthesia, 1995. **50**(3): p. 203-205.

130.   www.exatest.com, *Magnesium Deficiency - IntraCellular Diagnostics' EXAtest for Minerals Electrolytes*

131.   www.bodybio.com, *BodyBio Company*

132.   Durlach, J., et al., *Taurine and magnesium homeostasis: new data and recent advances.* Magnesium in cellular processes and medicine. Basel: S Karger publ, 1987: p. 219-38.

133.   www.douglaslabs.com, *Douglas Labs*

134.   www.selfhealthsystems.com, *Self-Health Systems - Magnesium Lotion*

135.   Shealy, C.N., *Holy Water, Sacred Oil.* 2000, Fair Grove, MO: Biogenics.

136.   Gaby, A.R., *Intravenous nutrient therapy: the "Myers' cocktail.".* Altern Med Rev, 2002. 7(5): p. 389-403.

137.   Turnlund, J.R., et al., *Vitamin B-6 depletion followed by repletion with animal-or plant-source diets and calcium and magnesium metabolism in young women.* Am J Clin Nutr, 1992. **56**(5): p. 905-10.

138.   Holman, P., *Pyridoxine–vitamin B-6.* Journal of the Australasian College of Nutritional and Environmental Medicine (ACNEM), 1995. **14**: p. 5-16.

139.   Schauss, A. and C. Costin, *Zinc as a nutrient in the treatment of eating disorders.* Am J Nat Med, 1997. **4**: p. 8-13.

140.   www.kirkmanlabs.com, *Kirkman Labs*

141.   www.realsalt.com, *RealSalt*

142.   Brownstein, D., *Salt Your Way to Health.* 2007: Medical Alternatives Press.

143.   www.thyroid.about.com, *Thyroid Disease Information*

144.   www.stopthethyroidmadness.com, *Stop The Thyroid Madness*

145.   Resnick, D. and G. Niwayama, *Diagnosis of Bone and Joint Disorders.* 1988: Philadelphia.

146.   Wald, A. and S.A. Adibi, *Stimulation of gastric acid secreted by glycine and related oligopeptides in humans.* American Journal of Physiology- Gastrointestinal and Liver Physiology, 1982. **242**(2): p. 85-88.

147.   Grobben, A.H., et al., *Inactivation of the bovine-spongiform-encephalopathy (BSE) agent by the acid and alkaline processes used in the manufacture of bone gelatine.* Biotechnology and Applied Biochemistry, 2004. **39**(3): p. 329-338.

148.   Prudden, J.F. and L.L. Balassa, *The biological activity of bovine cartilage preparations. Clinical demonstration of their potent anti-inflammatory capacity with supplementary notes on certain*

relevant fundamental supportive studies. Semin Arthritis Rheum, 1974. **3**(4): p. 287-321.

149. Samonina, G., et al., *Protection of gastric mucosal integrity by gelatin and simple proline-containing peptides.* Pathophysiology, 2000. **7**(1): p. 69-73.

150. Moskowitz, R.W., *Role of collagen hydrolysate in bone and joint disease.* Seminars in Arthritis and Rheumatism, 2000. **30**(2): p. 87-99.

151. www.greatlakesgelatin.com, *Great Lakes Gelatin, Grayslake, Illinois*

152. Yehuda, S. and R. Carasso, *Modulation of learning, pain thresholds, and thermoregulation in the rat by preparations of free purified alpha-linolenic and linoleic acids: determination of the optimal omega 3-to-omega 6 ratio.* Proc Natl Acad Sci US A, 1993. **90**(21): p. 10345-10349.

153. Erasmus, U., *Fats that heal, fats that kill.* 1993: Alive Books.

154. Hansen, A.E., et al., *ROLE OF LINOLEIC ACID IN INFANT NUTRITION: Clinical and Chemical Study of 428 Infants Fed on Milk Mixtures Varying in Kind and Amount of Fat.* Pediatrics, 1963. **31**(1): p. 171-192.

155. Daley, C.A., et al., *A Literature Review of the Value-Added Nutrients found in Grass-fed Beef Products,* College of Agriculture, California State University, Chico.

156. www.christophereggs.com, *Christopher Eggs*

157. Milinsk, M.C., et al., *Fatty acid profile of egg yolk lipids from hens fed diets rich in n-3 fatty acids.* Food Chemistry, 2003. **83**(2): p. 287-292.

158. Gower, J.D., *A role for dietary lipids and antioxidants in the activation of carcinogens.* Free Radical Biology & Medicine, 1988. **5**(2): p. 95-111.

159. Mozaffarian, D., E.B. Rimm, and D.M. Herrington, *Dietary fats, carbohydrate, and progression of coronary atherosclerosis in postmenopausal women.* American Journal of Clinical Nutrition, 2004. **80**(5): p. 1175-1184.

160. Fujiyama-Fujiwara, Y., et al., *Effects of sesamin on the fatty acid composition of the liver of rats fed N-6 and N-3 fatty acid-rich diet.* J Nutr Sci Vitaminol (Tokyo), 1995. **41**(2): p. 217-25.

161.   Shimizu, S., et al., *Sesamin is a potent and specific inhibitor of delta-5 desaturase in polyunsaturated fatty acid biosynthesis.* Lipids, 1991. **26**(7): p. 512-516.

162.   Wagner, S. and H. Breiteneder, *The latex-fruit syndrome.* Biochem Soc Trans, 2002. **30**(pt 6): p. 935-940.

163.   Fernandez-Rivas, M., R. van Ree, and M. Cuevas, *Allergy to Rosaceae fruits without related pollinosis.* J Allergy Clin Immunol, 1997. **100**(6 Pt 1): p. 728-33.

164.   Wright, J. and L. Lenard, *Why Stomach Acid Is Good for You.* 2001, M. Evans and Company.

165.   www.twinlab.com, *Twinlab Supplements*

166.   www.standardprocess.com, *Standard Process*

167.   Alverdy, J.C., *The re-emerging role of the intestinal microflora in critical illness and inflammation.* J Leukoc Biol, 2007: p. 1-6.

168.   Mitsou, E.K., et al., *Fecal microflora of Greek healthy neonates.* Anaerobe, 2007.

169.   Gibson, G.R. and R.A. Rastall, *When we eat, which bacteria should we be feeding.* ASM News, 2004. **70**: p. 224-231.

170.   Vogel, G., *CLINICAL TRIALS: Deaths Prompt a Review of Experimental Probiotic Therapy.* Science, 2008. **319**(5863): p. 557a-.

171.   Rodenburg, W., et al., *Impaired barrier function by dietary fructo-oligosaccharides (FOS) in rats is accompanied by increased colonic mitochondrial gene expression.* BMC Genomics, 2008. **9**(1): p. 144.

172.   Kirsch, M., *Bacterial overgrowth.* American Journal of Gastroenterology, 1990. **85**(3): p. 231-237.

173.   Bouhnik, Y., et al., *Bacterial populations contaminating the upper gut in patients with small intestinal bacterial overgrowth syndrome.* The American Journal of Gastroenterology, 1999. **94**(5): p. 1327-1331.

174.   www.kyolic.com, *Wakunaga -Kyolic Brand*

175.   Majamaa, H. and E. Isolauri, *Probiotics: a novel approach in the management of food allergy.* J Allergy Clin Immunol, 1997. **99**(2): p. 179-85.

176.   Lewis, W.H. and M.P.F. Elvin-Lewis, *Medical Botany: Plants Affecting Human Health.* 2003: Wiley.

177.   Odenyo, A.A. and P.O. Osuji, *Tannin-tolerant ruminal bacteria from East African ruminants.* Canadian Journal of Microbiology, 1998. **44**: p. 905-909.

178.   Jones, R.J. and R.G. Megarrity, *Successful transfer of DHP-degrading bacteria from Hawaiian goats to Australian ruminants to overcome the toxicity of Leucaena.* Aust Vet J, 1986. **63**(8): p. 259-62.

179.   www.terrapond.com, *Terramin Clay*

INDEX

LaVergne, TN USA
19 August 2009
155283LV00003B/8/P